GASTROINTESTINAL ENDOS
AND RELATED PROCEDURES

A Handbook for Nurses and Assistants

GASTROINTESTINAL ENDOSCOPY AND RELATED PROCEDURES

A Handbook for Nurses and Assistants

Morag M. Ravenscroft
Sister in Charge

and

Charles H. J. Swan
Consultant Physician
Department of Gastroenterology
City General Hospital
Stoke-on-Trent

LONDON
CHAPMAN AND HALL

First published 1984
by Chapman and Hall Ltd
11 New Fetter Lane, London EC4P 4EE

Printed in Great Britain at
the University Press, Cambridge

ISBN 0 412 24180 3 (hbk)
ISBN 0 412 16600 3 (pbk)

British Library Cataloguing in Publication Data

Ravenscroft, Morag M.
    Gastrointestinal endoscopy and related
    procedures.
    1. Endoscope and endoscopy
    2. Alimentary canal
    I. Title   II. Swan, Charles H. J.
    616.3'307545   RC804.E6

ISBN 0–412–24180–3
ISBN 0–412–16600–3 Pbk

CONTENTS

Dedicated to our friends in gastroenterology worldwide, who have been a constant source of stimulation and encouragement to us, both in production of this book and in our everyday clinical practice.

FOREWORD

Ever since the invention of the fiberoptic endoscope in 1888, gastrointestinal endoscopy has grown increasingly popular in day-to-day patient management. Most recently, a variety of therapeutic procedures are also being performed through the endoscope. With increasing technological advances, new endoscopic procedures will be appearing on the horizon. It, therefore, becomes extremely relevant for the gastrointestinal nurse or assistant to be familiar with various endoscopic procedures.

Gastrointestinal Endoscopy and Related Procedures will be a useful and practical guide in the making of a qualified gastrointestinal assistant. This book is notable for its elegant style, illustrations, detailed account of procedures, and especially the instructions on patient care. Discussions on physical preparation of gastrointestinal procedures, helpful hints and instrument care add to the value of this book. The psychological impact on the patient undergoing endoscopic procedures and the nurse's role in alleviating 'the fear of the unknown' also is properly covered in the text.

It is refreshing to see a nursing perspective in the writing of this text. Throughout the whole book, one can feel a warm and humane approach towards patients with gastrointestinal disease. All these and more are, of course, a result of Sister Morag Ravenscroft's vast experience along with the guidance of Dr Charles Swan.

It is a textbook worth reading and relishing.

Marcia Pfeifer R.N.
Former President of the SGA
Now with Gastroenterology Consultants Ltd,
Racine, Wis. USA

PREFACE

'Some books are to be tasted, others to be swallowed and some few to be chewed and digested.'

Francis Bacon
1561–1626

In planning the reading diet of students on our first Joint Board of Clinical Nursing Studies Short Course in Nursing for Gastrointestinal Endoscopy and Related Procedures (JBCNS No. 906), it became apparent that there was a shortage of books which provided a comprehensive reading background to this essentially practical training course.

This book represents a positive desire of the authors to pass on their knowledge and experience in gastroenterology to nurses, and perhaps doctors, who are working in this fast developing specialist medical field. It seemed a natural development for both authors who have for some time been involved in teaching the subject to doctors and nurses.

Although designed primarily for qualified nurses involved in diagnostic gastroenterology and therapeutic endoscopy, it may also be used as a reference book by student nurses, ward staff and medical students.

Most books on this subject have been written by doctors and the role of the nurse in gastroenterology has been defined by the clinicians. This book gives a change of emphasis and provides a balance of anatomy and physiology, applied pathology and the rationale behind the diagnostic and therapeutic procedures with particular reference to nursing care. It defines the professional role of the nurse in the gastroenterology department, providing guidelines for the management, research and teaching involvement likely to be incurred. It also includes a comprehensive section on the structure and care of instruments, aimed to ensure a high standard of technique to prevent damage to instruments, costly repairs and cross infection.

This book does not describe nursing care of ward patients suffering from gastroenterological problems but seeks to complement other texts which describe medical or surgical nursing care.

It is hoped that by writing this book, we will have further advanced the quality of care of the patient and helped increase nurses' satisfaction from their work in this absorbing and fascinating field. We hope the book reflects the immense personal pleasure and satisfaction both authors enjoy in their field of work.

M.M.R.
C.H.J.S.

ACKNOWLEDGEMENTS

We would like to thank our colleagues for their helpful comments on the manuscript, Sister Anne Lloyd from Shrewsbury for her advice on the section on laparoscopy and Sister Joy Pollard for information on bowel preparation prior to colonoscopy. Our thanks also to the Departments of Medical Photography and Drug Information Service, North Staffordshire Health Authority for their invaluable assistance and to the Staff of the Department of Gastroenterology for their understanding during the period of writing this book. The equipment companies who provided information were ACM Endoscopy, GMI Medical Ltd, KeyMed Ltd, Macarthys, Medisco, Medoc (Glos.) Ltd, and Pyser Ltd and we are very grateful for their contributions.

Our special thanks go to Christopher Davies for the illustrations and to Carol Higginson for her constant secretarial support and forbearance.

We are indebted to the Endoscopy Committee of the British Society of Gastroenterology who gave their permission for inclusion of Appendix A 'Endoscopy and infection'.

1

ROLE OF THE NURSE

INTRODUCTION

'A trained nurse is the ideal person to assist in the organisation of an endoscopy service and at the actual examination.'

BSDE Memorandum, 1973

The nurse entering a specialized field such as gastroenterology should have at least one year's post-registration experience which will have given her the opportunity to develop her nursing skills, exposed her to first line management experience and enabled her to bring a mature approach to the specialty. It is important that a nurse in a relatively new and specialized field does not become isolated. It is also imperative that she receives training in the subject and is allowed contact with sources of information and education which will help her to develop her job to the benefit of the patient and to increase her job satisfaction.

The British Society of Gastroenterology Endoscopy Assistants Group and the Society of Gastrointestinal Assistants in the USA provide membership for nurses and assistants in the field of endoscopy and gastroenterology nursing. A newsletter is published regularly and personal contact with other nurses through meetings and conferences can be of great value. In the UK, the Royal College of Nursing seeks to promote the education of the nurse in gastro-enterology and give recognition to her professional status in this clinical specialty. The Joint Board of Clinical Nursing Studies developed a short course for nurses in gastroenterology in 1979 covering the aspects of the work contained in this book. The course runs for 10–13 days and is the only recognized form of post-registration training in the UK. The course is 50% theoretical and 50% practical and a certificate of attendance is issued to all who complete the course. From 1983 this course will continue under the aegis of the UK Central Council for Nurses and Midwives. In the USA the Society of Gastrointestinal Assistants run a variety of courses.

The duties of the nurse in gastroenterology are:

Patient care
Instrument care
Management
Teaching/research

PATIENT CARE

The nurse is primarily responsible for the care of the patient, the physical and psychological preparation for all investigations and treatment, care during the procedures and after-care prior to discharge of the patient home or into the care of other ward staff for overnight or longer term stay. A qualified nurse already has sufficient knowledge of the general nursing care of the patient undergoing investigative or therapeutic gastroenterological procedures. She should be familiar with the anatomy and physiology of the gastrointestinal tract in order to understand the procedures and so that she can prepare the patient physically and psychologically.

Physical preparation

For most investigations and therapeutic procedures of the gastrointestinal tract, the organ involved must be empty and free from residual food and debris. Specific instructions are given for the physical preparation required for each procedure under the appropriate chapter headings.

Psychological preparation

It is essential, in order to carry out a satisfactory procedure, that the patient is prepared psychologically to accept the physical aspects of the procedure. Any investigation or treatment is a form of assault of the body and can cause resistance and embarrassment should the patient be unable to understand the reasons for the procedure and if the procedure is carried out in a manner or atmosphere lacking in reassurance. In order to retain the patient's confidence, a good relationship between doctor, nurse and patient should be established at the earliest opportunity. An explanation of the problem giving rise to the need for the test or treatment is best given direct to the patient by the doctor who has the clinical responsibility. The nurse receiving the patient will need to reassure herself that the patient has understood the explanation and if necessary give some added advice.

Most gastrointestinal procedures involve the passage of a tube, and it should be explained to the patient that they may have to swallow a tube with assistance from the doctor and/or nurse and that local anaesthetic and sedation will help make this easier. Any discomfort felt will be temporary and inevitable and will probably be forgotten because of the sedation. Large bowel investigation requires a different approach since a major effect on the patient may be to cause embarrassment as well as discomfort. Reassurance from the nurse and privacy during the procedure are important to ensure the patient's co-operation and confidence.

Care during procedures

The nurse's duties during endoscopic and other gastrointestinal procedures cover the physical safety and psychological well-being of the patient. By ensuring correctly functioning equipment, the provision of adequate facilities, the availability of correct drugs and resuscitation facilities, the physical aspects of care can be ensured. In order to ensure the psychological well-being of the patient, the nurse is required to understand the purpose and technique of the procedure to which the patient is being subjected. It is then necessary for her to explain the procedure to the patient in terms which can be understood. Only then, can any procedure be carried out safely with the full co-operation of the patient.

Upper gastrointestinal procedures

During upper gastrointestinal procedures, the nurse must be aware of the hazards likely to arise from the actual procedure and the drugs involved. The nurse is able to observe the patient's vital functions while the doctor is involved with the view down the endoscope or while he is carrying out any investigative or therapeutic procedure. She should observe the patient's pulse, respiration rate and colour and maintain him in the correct position throughout the procedure. This facilitates ease of examination and adds safety and comfort for the patient. She must maintain the patient's airway by careful and discriminate use of suction and should reassure the patient throughout the procedure. Usually, sedation will make the patient relaxed and drowsy but not un-conscious, and it is essential that the nurse remembers to treat the patient appropriately with carefully chosen words of explanation whilst ensuring that conversation in the room is kept to a minimum.

Lower gastrointestinal procedures

Sedation may be used in some lower bowel investigations and care of the sedated patient is essential. Observation of pulse, blood pressure, respiration rate and colour, plus reassurance and a quiet atmosphere are essential. The door is best kept closed to ensure privacy and to prevent waiting and recovering patients from seeing or hearing what is going on in the endoscopy room. Check blood pressure before procedure (i.e. after bowel preparation). Once again, position is important during lower bowel examinations as this helps to ensure a safe and satisfactory procedure. The nurse will be responsible for maintaining the correct position and ensuring that the patient is as comfortable as possible.

After care

Upper gastrointestinal procedures

The general principles of the care of the sedated patient are applied. It is essential that the patient is fully conscious and has a satisfactory swallowing reflex. Care must be taken that the effects of any local anaesthetic have worn off before food and drink are given. Explanation that most abdominal discomfort is due to the insufflation of air and that this will gradually lessen should be given. Particular problems relating to some procedures are dealt with in the appropriate chapters.

Lower gastrointestinal procedures

The care of the sedated patient again applies. The nurse should ensure that the patient is clean, dry and comfortable while recovering from the procedure and may again need to reassure the patient that any discomfort will soon pass. Special reference is made to particular problems under the appropriate section.

The patient should be discharged from the unit with the knowledge that the procedure was carried out satisfactorily and with such information about the result as the doctor and nurse consider relevant.

MANAGEMENT

The nursing management of a gastroenterology department depends on the range of service provided, the number of staff employed and the line management position of the individual nurse involved. In order to cope with the service provided it is essential to ensure that there are sufficient staff to cover holidays, study days, sickness and work taking place outside the department. For example, a nurse may be assisting at a session in the Radiology department.

The Gastroenterology service in a District General Hospital should provide:

Upper gastrointestinal endoscopy
'Bleeder' service
Colonoscopy and polypectomy
Endoscopic retrograde cholangiopancreatography

Non-endoscopic procedures such as:

Secretion tests
Malabsorption investigations
Liver biopsy

may also be catered for and will require sufficient nursing and technical staff.

A suggested staff structure for a department providing the above service is as follows:

SRN – Sister Grade II
Additional nursing staff: Staff nurse(s)
State enrolled nurse(s)
Clerical/secretarial personnel
Nursing auxiliary
Orderly

Liaison

The nurse in charge of the department will be required to liaise with other hospital departments in order to guarantee the smooth running of the department. Contact with the Radiology department, wards, administrators, hospital medical personnel, stores, domestic and maintenance personnel will all fall within the responsibility of the gastroenterology nurse. She should develop good interdepartmental relationships and learn whom she should contact to solve problems within her department.

One of the most important contacts the nurse working in endoscopy will need to make and consolidate at an early stage in her appointment will be with the appropriate instrument companies. Local arrangements for the repair and maintenance of equipment must be observed, but the nurse should form a relationship with instrument companies in order to gain information and advice about the endoscopy equipment and accessories under her care. The companies play a vital part in helping to maintain a good service to the patient by providing information leaflets, rapid servicing and repair facilities and useful advice by telephone and directly from their representatives in the field.

The day to day organization of the department will depend on the efficiency of the nurse in charge. She may be responsible for:

Organizing lists
Sending appointments to patients
Arranging the provision of the 'emergency' endoscopy service
Liaising with wards for the treatment of inpatients and for the provision of beds for patients who may require to be admitted from the department
Ensuring satisfactory documentation of all procedures carried out in the department
Photographic records
Recording of pathology specimens obtained – the forms, containers and department record book
Liaising with the Radiology department for screening time for procedures where necessary

INSTRUMENT CARE

That component of the role of the gastroenterology nurse which may be completely new to her is the technical knowledge necessary to maintain the equipment involved. It is essential that early training is given in the structure, function, cleaning and disinfection, maintenance and repairs of all equipment and accessories in the nurse's care. Without clean, functioning equipment it will be impossible to provide an efficient service to the patient. This training can be provided by the instrument companies, by visits to other units and by approved training courses. A great deal of the training will inevitably be in-service training and help should be available to the nurse from other nurses in post, medical personnel, nurse managers and teachers. Representatives of the instrument companies are also helpful in providing information and demonstrations of equipment in their product range.

The structure, care, cleaning and disinfection of instruments is covered in Chapter 2.

TEACHING AND RESEARCH

It is part of the duty of every qualified nurse to pass on her knowledge to colleagues and learners. Opportunities to learn how to teach arise via management courses and in-service training departments and expert advice is readily available.

Nurses in specialized areas such as gastroenterology have a responsibility to ensure that other hospital nurses can gain as much knowledge as possible while visiting the specialized department. The nurse in charge may also be involved in talking to groups of trained staff about her work, thus helping to improve the care of patients and develop good relations with wards and departments throughout the hospital.

Should the service and the expertise of the gastroenterology staff make it possible, the nurse may be involved in training nurses in this specific field. Liaison with nurse education staff will ensure the nurse has the support and confidence to teach her subject satisfactorily.

Research is an ongoing process within many units and may cover clinical trials, drug trials and nursing research. It is often the nurse who is a permanent member of the research team and it is helpful if she is involved in the planning and setting up of trials within her department. Clinical and drug trials require careful structuring to avoid interference with the every day running of the department. The trial must be accepted by the local ethical committee and should be part of the general care of the patient. Clinical drug trials will involve the monitoring of patients' response to treatment and may include such things as venepuncture, questionnaires and diaries of symptoms and drugs taken.

The department nurse can assist with the collection of such information after suitable training.

Nursing research is required to evaluate the nurse's role, to record the efficiency of nursing staff and to help plan staff structures within a department.

Documentation

As in other clinical areas, careful records are required for inclusion in the patient's case notes and in the department files. These are often used retrospectively for research and planning purposes. The most common types of letters and reports which may be required are:

Letter of appointment: specifying date and time, plus clear instructions as to the location of the department. Warnings must be given on the letter about the effects of sedation and if necessary, about the likely exposure to radiation.

Consent form: giving details of the procedure to be carried out. This form can be a routine hospital operation consent form or forms can be specifically designed for each type of gastroenterology procedure.

Medicine sheet: a record of drugs administered is also required for the case notes.

Report form: on completion of each procedure, a report on the findings must be completed. This will include the patient's name, case note number, date of birth etc. and various types of report forms are available.

Records of orders for ancillary equipment, the working condition of endoscopes and the repair history of equipment will also be important for the efficient running of the department.

Photography

The photographic recording of endoscopic findings contributes to:

Improved documentation of the patient's clinical condition
Good teaching facilities within the department
Extra research sources

The methods of photographic recording can be:

Transparencies
Prints
Video

Photographic methods are dealt with in greater depth in Chapter 2.

2

FACILITIES FOR GASTROINTESTINAL INVESTIGATIONS

ENDOSCOPES

History

The gastrointestinal tract was first inspected by rigid instruments. Hippocrates is recorded as having inspected the rectum with a candle, whilst more recently a rigid sigmoidoscope was used by Bozzini in 1795. The stomach had to wait nearly a century to be viewed directly. At that time, von Mickulicz-Radicki, building on the earlier efforts of Kussmaul, finally achieved a successful inspection of the stomach in 1881. Rigid sigmoidoscopes and proctoscopes still have a very important role in the inspection of the rectal and distal colonic mucosa, but rigid gastroscopes have been supplanted by fibreoptic instruments. The development of fibreoptic instruments has occurred in the past twenty years and adoption for routine use in most district general hospitals has been largely due to their simplicity, ease of use and safety for the patient.

Professor Harold Hopkins of Reading University, UK, deserves the credit for developing some early work of John Logie Baird, the inventor of television, to design useable fibreoptic bundles. In the early 1950s Hopkins produced fibreoptic bundles which would faithfully transmit an image. The optical principles involved depend on total internal reflection of light within each fibre (Fig. 2.1). To facilitate this, each fibre is coated with a glass of low refractive index before the fibres are bound together into a bundle. The fibre bundles are of two types: (1) non-coherent bundles which are satisfactory for conduction of light but do not give a satisfactory image, and (2) coherent bundles which, on the other hand, are so optically perfect that what is looked at one end of the bundle may be faithfully reproduced at the other (Fig. 2.2). It is the use of these principles which is behind the fibreoptic instrument as we know it today.

Every modern flexible instrument has the same basic features whether it be a gastroscope, duodenoscope or colonoscope. Dependent upon its basic purpose,

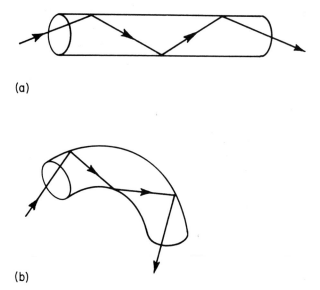

(a)

(b)

Fig. 2.1   *The properties of fibreglass filaments. (a) Total internal reflection, (b) light can travel round corners.*

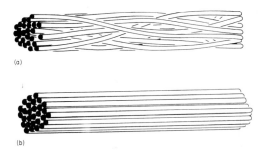

(a)

(b)

Fig. 2.2   *The difference between (a) non-coherent and (b) coherent fibreglass bundles.*

it will be end-viewing (oesophagoscope, gastroscope, colonoscope) or side-viewing (duodenoscope). Attempts to combine the features of both end- and side-viewing instruments have been successfully fulfilled in a versatile forward/oblique viewing instrument.

Structure

The construction of each instrument is such that it has an optical system consisting of the following:

At least one fibre bundle of the non-coherent type to conduct light to the stomach (called the light guide)

A fibre bundle to conduct the image to the eye (called the image guide)

A system of lenses to focus the image at the eye-piece.

A control head in which is housed the lenses, levers to control the flexible tip and buttons or switches to control suction or airflow through the instrument

An insertion tube. This is the part which enters the patient. It is of variable length, usually from one to two metres. It is of special construction being extremely flexible, whilst at the same time sturdy and waterproof. Its basic design is of metal inner layers rather like flexible gas-piping and a vinyl outer sheath. Inside the insertion tube are packed the air/water flow channel, suction channel, the wires which control movement of the flexible tip, the light guides and the image guide (Figs 2.3 and 2.4).

Such is the design of an instrument that these features can all be packed into an instrument of about 1 cm in diameter whilst still maintaining flexibility.

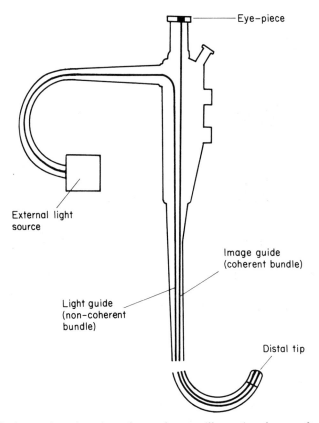

Fig. 2.3   *The internal construction of an endoscope illustrating the use of coherent and non-coherent fibre bundles.*

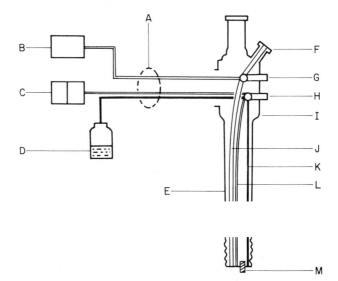

Fig. 2.4   *Internal construction of an endoscope showing suction and air–water channel arrangements. A, endoscope umbilical; B, suction pump; C, air pump; D, water reservoir; E, endoscope insertion tube; F, biopsy port; G, suction button; H, air/wash button; I, endoscope control head; J, combined suction/biopsy channel; K, water channel; L, air channel; M, combined air/water port.*

The flexible tip has four-way angulation controlled by wires which run all the way through the insertion tube (Fig. 2.5). They are attached at the very end of the flexible tip and are controlled by the levers on the control head. Up–down movement is controlled by one lever and right–left movement is controlled by the other. The design of modern instrument is such that the flexibility if often in excess of 180° in each direction. Combination of use of the two levers allows polydirectional tip movement. The position of the tip can be held in a fixed position by a special brake facility built into the lever system on the control head.

Inspection of the tip of the instrument will reveal all the features so far described; namely the extreme flexibility, suction channel, image and light guides and the air delivery supplies. The suction channel doubles as a biopsy channel and it is down this that instruments such as biopsy forceps, cytology brushes or diathermy snares can be passed. The air delivery nipples are usually arranged in such a way that they can act as lens cleaners. This facility is also controlled from the head of the instrument and means that a jet of water can be squirted over the face of the distal tip, thereby cleaning debris away from the surface to improve vision (Fig. 2.6).

All of these features make up the 'working parts' of the endoscope. It has to be connected to services such as light, suction and air supply. Modern instruments are designed such that these connections are made through a single connecting tube or umbilical which comes off the side of the control head of

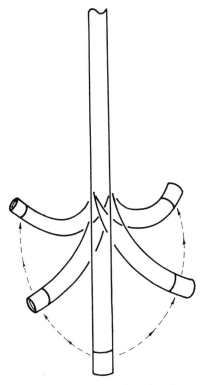

Fig. 2.5 *Distal tip of instrument showing polydirectional movement capability.*

the instrument. It too, has extreme flexibility and is usually over one metre in length. Inspection of its end reveals a complicated system of connections which join up with air, water and suction at a light source conveniently housed in a compact cabinet. The small extra connections which can be seen at the end of the connecting tube are part of the control system for the camera/flash facility built into the instrument.

The powerful light system is housed in the source box, together with the air pump which provides inflation facilities. The water reservoir, which is part of the lens-cleaning system, is conveniently attached to the light source and joins the connecting tube by a simple air- and water-tight seal. Two other facilities may be located attached to the connecting tube close to the light source. One is an attachment for a diathermy connection, thereby effectively grounding the instrument to the diathermy source if appropriate. The other is a connection for a carbon dioxide supply. This facility is only provided on colonoscopes where insufflation of carbon dioxide is considered to be desirable to minimize the risk of explosions within the patient during diathermy. Under these circumstances, the carbon dioxide gas flow is controlled by a button located separately on the control head of the instrument.

The size of the light source will vary, dependent upon the purpose of the endoscopy. Standard procedures in the upper gastrointestinal tract and the colon can usually be carried out with adequate illumination from quite a small light source in which is housed a halogen filament bulb of the halogen reflector

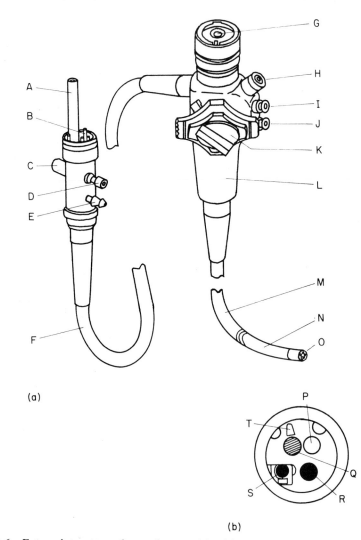

(a)

(b)

Fig. 2.6 *External structure of an endoscope (a), with an expanded view of the distal tip (b). A, light guide connection; B, air pump connection; C, suction pump connection; D, diathermy earth connection; E, suction pump connection; F, umbilical connecting endoscope to light source and services; G, eye-piece; H, biopsy port; I, suction button; J, air/water button; K, control wheels for up/down and lateral tip movement; L, control head; M, insertion tube; N, bending section; O, distal tip; P, image guide; Q, light guide; R, biopsy/suction channel; S, forceps raiser; T, wash jet.*

type. Within the cabinet will also be housed a fan-cooling system for the bulb and a simple air pump already mentioned. The circuitry is protected by a simple fuse. Inspection of the face of the light source reveals the connections of the umbilical of the endoscope, an on/off switch and a control for intensity of light. Some light sources have a switch which controls intermittency of air supply.

If closed circuit television or cine-photography using the endoscope is planned then this simple light source will be inadequate. In these circumstances, a much more powerful light source with a xenon lamp will be necessary. Whilst producing a light of greater intensity, these powerful light sources still incorporate the same basic connections for air, water and suction. The reader is advised to consult the manufacturers' literature for the specification of the various light sources available.

Various accessories are available for use with all instruments. Some form part of the basis of an endoscopy service, whilst others are used in more advanced endoscopic techniques.

One of the major benefits of endoscopy over radiology is the opportunity to take biopsies for histological assessment of lesions. These biopsy forceps can be passed down the suction channel of the endoscope and are colour and size-coded

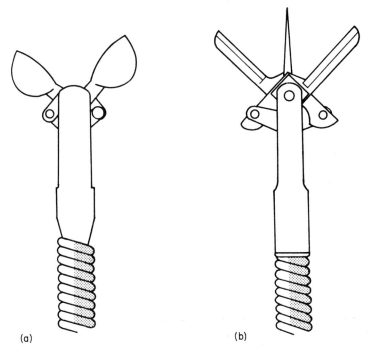

(a)   (b)

Fig. 2.7 Biopsy forceps. (a) Standard cupped forceps and (b) spiked forceps.

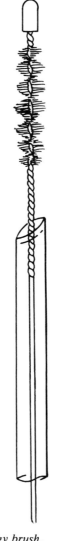

Fig. 2.8   *Sheathed disposable cytology brush.*

for a specific instrument. The commonest type is simple cupped forceps, but elongated or even fenestrated types are available. The addition of a central spike can be very beneficial when trying to obtain biopsies from a site where only a glancing approach can be made (Fig. 2.7).

Extra information about the nature of some lesions can be obtained with brush cytology, but this is very dependent on local cytology services, since not all hospitals have a department which can take on the added work-load of gastrointestinal cytology. Various brushes are available but the best type is the

sheathed brush in which the tiny brush is protected by a plastic sheath. After
harvesting cells from a suspect lesion, the head of the brush is withdrawn into
the outer sheath before removal from the endoscope. This has the advantage of

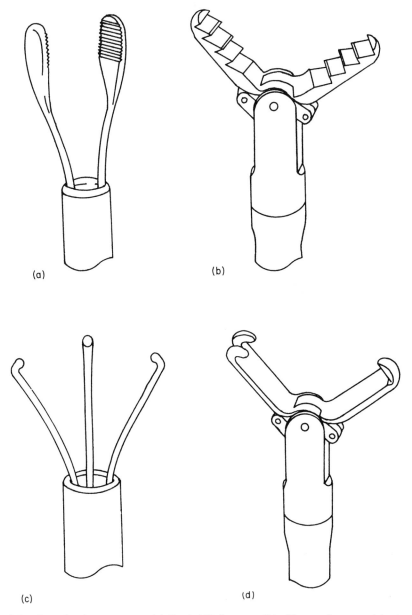

(a)

(b)

(c)

(d)

Fig. 2.9 *Grasping instruments. (a) Duck-bill forceps, (b) alligator forceps, (c) tripod
forceps and (d) rat-toothed forceps.*

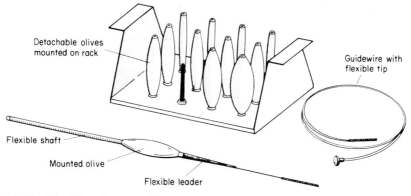

Fig. 2.10   *The Eder–Puestow dilators.*

minimizing the shedding of cells into the suction/biopsy channel, thereby reducing the risk of false positive results. Although sold as disposable brushes, most types are reusable for three or four times, after diligent cleaning of the bristles and resterilization by autoclaving (Fig. 2.8).

Various grasping or retrieval devices are also available. These range from polyp-graspers through a variety of different-jawed forceps used for the retrieval of foreign bodies such as coins, razor blades and pins. It is probably advisable to have one of these devices available should the request for foreign body removal be made (Fig. 2.9). Also available are tiny scissors used for cutting retained non-absorbable sutures which can be visualized occasionally.

A major simple advance in the range of therapeutic procedures conducted with endoscopes is the dilatation of benign oesophageal strictures. These seem to occur most commonly in elderly patients in whom repeated general anaesthesia and rigid oesophagoscopy represents a serious hazard. A safe alternative is the use of the Eder–Puestow dilators with an end-viewing fibreoptic instrument. The system consists of a long guide-wire, two flexible wands and a series of olives of increasing size which may be threaded onto the wands (Fig. 2.10). An alternative is to use the recently developed Celestin stepped dilator (Fig. 2.11).

An extension to this technique of benign dilatation is the palliation of inoperable malignant strictures by dilatation and the insertion of a tube pros-thesis. This may be achieved using the Nottingham tube introducer which incorporates an expanding device to grip the inside of the prosthesis (Fig. 2.12) or the Medoc system which is dependent on a Mandril system or a balloon inflated within the tube (Fig. 2.13).

The use of these devices is described in greater detail in Chapter 3.

If endoscopic polypectomy is to be undertaken, then a diathermy system will be necessary. This consists of a diathermy generator active lead which may be connected to forceps, snares or bulb-ended electrodes, a patient plate and its connecting lead and an attachment to earth the endoscope. This type of system

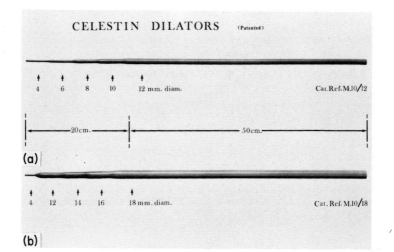

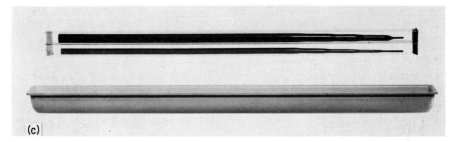

Fig. 2.11 Celestin thermoplastic stepped dilators. (a) 12 mm diameter; (b) 18 mm diameter; (c) two dilators in cooling baths ready for use. (Courtesy of Medoc (Glos) Ltd.)

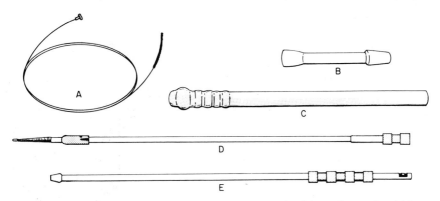

Fig. 2.12 Nottingham oesophageal tube introducer. A, flexible guidewire; B, Atkinson tube; C, rammer; D, inner shaft with expansile olive; E, outer shaft.

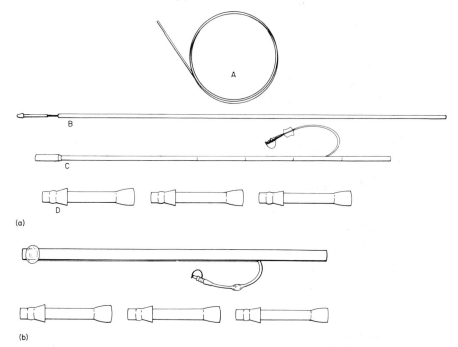

Fig. 2.13 *(a) Mandril set for oesophageal intubation using Medoc flanged tube. A, guide wire; B, Mandril; C, inflatable balloon introducer; D, Medoc flanged tubes. (b) Over-endoscope insertion tube for oesophageal intubation using Medoc flanged tube.*

is usually designed to deliver cutting or coagulating current to the polyp snare but recent work suggests that blended current containing a mixture of cutting/coagulating current may have some advantages. The same type of system will be required for endoscopic sphincterotomy for removal of common bile duct stones. This type of diathermy system is called monopolar, not to be confused with a bipolar system which has some potential for the coagulation of bleeding lesions (Fig. 2.14). It is strongly recommended that the manufacturer's specifications be considered before an appropriate diathermy source is obtained.

When the most suitable diathermy equipment/supply unit has been chosen, then appropriate snares may be purchased. It is important that their connections match the equipment/supply unit. Snares are of simple construction, consisting of an insulated handle and outer sleeve, down which runs a braided wire which is formed into a loop at the lower end where it passes out of the insulated section. The loop can be formed into a variety of shapes and can vary in size. Popular shapes are a simple oval, hexagon or 'D' shape. Whilst readily available from instrument manufacturers, some endoscopists prefer to make their own snares. This is perfectly safe provided the insulation facility is observed. If not, then electric current may leak through to the endoscope and may burn the patient or the endoscopist.

The same construction principles apply to endoscopic papillotomes. Once again, these have an insulated handle and outer sleeve with appropriate connections to a diathermy unit/source. In this case, the distal wire of the device, which is used for cutting into and enlarging the papilla of Vater at the lower end of the common bile duct, is shaped into a single strand of wire. It may be used to cut open the papilla, thereby aiding the removal of gallstones from the duct.

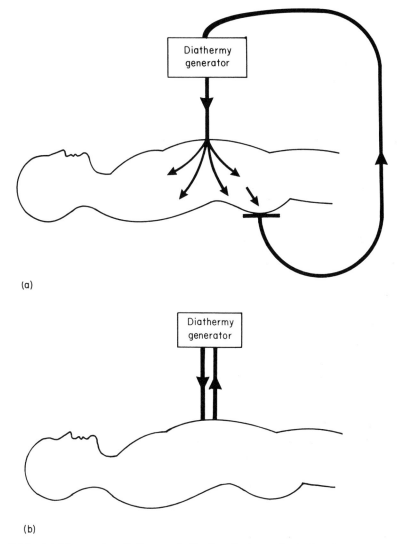

Fig. 2.14 *(a) Monopolar diathermy, indicating that a patient plate is necessary since energy passes through the body of the patient before returning to the diathermy generator. (b) Bipolar diathermy, indicating that a patient plate is not required since current returns to the generator via a single electrode.*

One of the more recent developments in fibreoptic endoscopy has been the use of a long flexible needle introduced down the biopsy channel. It is particularly valuable for injecting sclerosant solutions into oesophageal varices but could be used to inject other solutions into lesions elsewhere. It consists of an upper end with a Luer connection for syringe attachment, a long outer sheath of coiled wire construction and an inner core which is, in effect, a very long needle. The inner core may be withdrawn into the outer sleeve for safety during insertion but then may be extended at the moment of injection. The coiled wire construction makes these fragile accessories very difficult to clean. They are available in a variety of sizes to suit various endoscopes.

Another recent development is the application of laser light energy via the endoscope. A laser is a device for generating a high energy light beam. This beam can now be focused down a delivery system which is flexible and small enough to pass down the endoscope biopsy channel. Its principle use is in coagulating bleeding sources within the gastrointestinal tract. The two types of laser which have application in gastroenterology are the Argon laser and the Neodymium/YAG laser. Each emits energy of different wave length and therefore have differing applications. It has not yet been concluded which will prove the most versatile for endoscopic use. Built-in safety factors now ensure that unlimited energy may not be applied and that which is applied is only delivered when all conditions are in a safe state.

The valuable instruments, light sources and suction equipment described above are best used in conjunction with a purpose-designed endoscopy trolley. This means that all endoscopy facilities can be concentrated in a tidy manner rather than clutter floor space with a number of different trollies for various accessories. Endoscope trollies have built-in facilities to accommodate:

Light source
Suction unit
Biopsy forceps
Diathermy snares
Drugs, syringes and needles
Storage drawers

One of the most important features is the elevated edge to the trolley-top working surface. This has eliminated the risk of an instrument sliding to the floor from a non-lipped trolley top. The endoscopy trolley usually has a built-in block of power plugs so that a single connection may be made to the mains and all other electrical appliances may be connected directly at the trolley. This safety design feature reduces the number of trailing power cables (Fig. 2.15).

An important component of endoscopic practice is the teaching of techniques to trainee endoscopists. The assistant at endoscopy sessions will also gain added interest when able to visualize the procedure. The simplest method of doing so is to connect a teaching attachment or lecturescope to the observer end of the endoscope. The teaching attachment consists of a coherent fibre

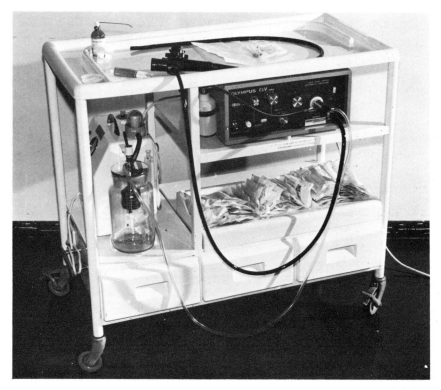

Fig. 2.15 *Endoscopy trolley set up ready for use.*

bundle, at one end of which is a locking attachment to align its optics with those of the endoscope and at the other end of which is an optical lens system to allow the observer to focus the endoscopic image. This is a simple but effective device to allow single observers to have a very good look at the endoscopic findings.

If observer groups are larger, a closed circuit television system (CCTV) should be considered. This consists of a beam-splitter which connects to the upper end of the endoscope, a televison camera and power unit and a monitor television screen on which the endoscopic findings are displayed. A video recording/play-back deck may also be incorporated into the system to increase its versatility. By this means, large groups can watch the endoscopic procedure simultaneously. The system has the benefit of recording endoscopic findings so that equivocal findings may be discussed at a later date or features preserved for case conference discussion.

Cleaning of small flexible accessories will be improved by the use of an ultrasonic cleaner. This consists of a small ultrasonic generator which connects to a water bath in which accessories can be immersed in detergent. The ultrasonic vibrations shake contaminating particles free from accessories in a manner which is impossible with simple brush cleaning. The accessories so cleaned may

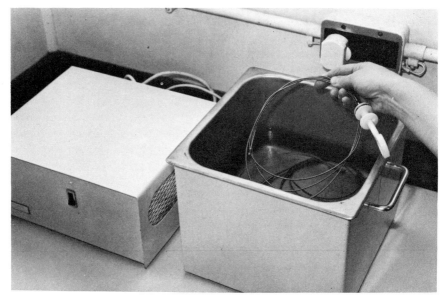

Fig. 2.16   *Ultrasonic cleaner.*

then be stored ready for use or dispatched for sterilization prior to reuse. The ultrasonic cleaning facility is particularly useful with accessories of coiled wire construction (Fig. 2.16).

Endoscopic photography

The facility to obtain good quality colour transparencies or photographic prints of endoscopically visualized lesions adds a further dimension to the usefulness of endoscopic practice. An accurate, permanent, visual record may be obtained of normal and abnormal appearances which may be of value in teaching, research and in the clinical record. Photographs are obtained by attaching to the eye-piece of the endoscope an appropriate camera, which has been previously loaded with the correct type of film. The technique is simplified by various semi-automatic processes within the equipment so that it is not necessary to be an expert photographer to obtain a good result. It is, however, necessary to observe certain guidelines with regard to light-source strength, film grade, exposure setting and camera shutter speed. All of this information is readily available from manufacturer's literature specific to the equipment purchased and is outside the scope of this book. Close adherence to the guidelines will ensure a good result (Fig. 2.17).

Most camera manufacturers produce single lens reflex cameras which can be adapted to endoscopic photography, but Fujinon, Pentax and Olympus companies all produce a range of adaptors which make their products the most acceptable. Olympus and Fujinon produce a 16 mm single lens reflex camera which is specifically developed for endoscopic work. It is lightweight and possesses a built-in motor advance of the film cassette. All of these cameras are usually used to produce colour transparencies of endoscopic findings.

For some time attempts have been made to adapt the Polaroid photographic principles to endoscopic use, and a very good quality Polaroid print can now be obtained instantaneously using the Polaroid Instant Endocamera model EC-3 and type 779 film. The major advantage of this system is that a colour print is available for storage and is especially useful for the clinical record. The major disadvantages are the extra cost of equipment and film and the need for a high

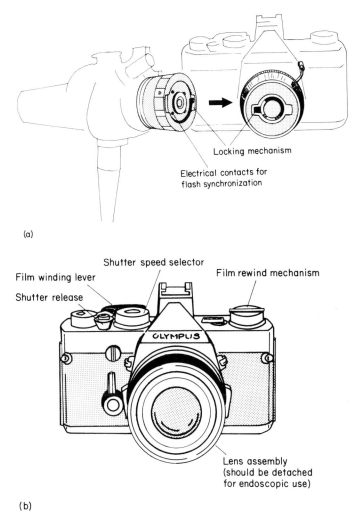

(a)

Locking mechanism

Electrical contacts for flash synchronization

Shutter speed selector

Film winding lever

Film rewind mechanism

Shutter release

OLYMPUS

Lens assembly (should be detached for endoscopic use)

(b)

Fig. 2.17 *(a) Endoscope eye-piece and camera with endoscope adaptor fitted, (b) A single-lens reflex camera suitable for endoscopic photography.*

intensity light source which is also more expensive than a routine light source. Colour prints for permanent record purposes can otherwise be obtained either as a print from a transparency by conventional photographic means or by the use of a new Polaroid Polaprinter. Each of these methods produces a permanent colour print, but the enlargement effect during the process results in a picture which lacks the definition of the original endoscopic view.

On a much more elaborate scale, cine-photography may be performed by attaching a cine camera to the eye-piece of the endoscope. It is unlikely that this facility will ever be part of routine practice and will be limited to those centres engaged in making teaching films of endoscopic technique. To an extent, the same is true of video films recorded during CCTV recording via the endoscope. CCTV is, however, a much simpler system to use and has additional benefits. Mobile arms have been developed to attach a lightweight television camera to the endoscope eye-piece via a beam-splitter. This enables the endoscopist to perform an endoscopy in the conventional manner whilst at the same time, allowing the television camera to receive an identical picture. This can then be transmitted to a television monitor screen and simultaneously recorded on a video deck. As a result, larger groups of observers have an opportunity to observe the endoscopic technique and findings and the result may be recorded for subsequent re-evaluation if required. No special photographic skills are required and the video tape is available for instant playback without a complex developing process or additional projection facilities. Although expensive, CCTV ought to be considered an essential item of equipment for any endoscopy unit regularly engaged in endoscopy teaching to groups rather than individuals whose needs may be fulfilled by a conventional fibreoptic teaching attachment. It is important to remember that both cine-photography and CCTV require a high intensity light source.

Guidelines for endoscopy assistants

Check list

Camera with film
Spare film
Film record book
Light source and camera settings: Shutter speed to '4' (i.e. ¼ second)
Shutter synchronization on camera set to 'X'
Camera set to 'manual'
Light source exposure index correctly set for unit and film grade (see manufacturer's literature)
Learn how to load and unload the film appropriate to the cameras available

continued

Know where to send the film for developing, which packaging to use and where to obtain fresh supplies

Maintain good liaison with the hospital photography department

Make sure that each patient's photographs are correctly identified either by photographing patient details in conjunction with the endoscopic photographs or by recording the details in a film record book, kept specially for the purpose. In it, for each film used, record:

Date film started
Patient details
Diagnosis
Frame numbers and number of photographs taken
Site and nature of lesion photographed
Date film completed and sent for processing
Date transparencies returned, mounted and stored

It is best to ask for return of the processed film in an unmounted strip. The transparencies can then be identified according to the film record book and may be cut, mounted and stored appropriately

With Polaroid prints, these should be mounted onto a card which bears the patient's clinical details. They may then pass directly into the clinical record

If the auto-exposure system fails, check and clean all electrical contacts on the camera and between the camera and the endoscope, and the endoscope and the light source

Always ensure that a camera is available wherever and whenever an endoscope is in use

Interesting pathology may be observed during any endoscopic procedure and the facility to record such findings should be instantly available

---

CARE OF ENDOSCOPES AND ACCESSORIES

The care of endoscopy equipment plays a vital part in the role of the endoscopy nurse. She must understand:

The purpose of the equipment
The structure of the equipment
The principles of cross infection in endoscopy
Understand how to clean, disinfect and maintain the equipment under her care

Fibreoptic endoscopes

All endoscopes require to be:

Functioning correctly

Clean and disinfected before use
The correct endoscope for the procedure
Maintained regularly

To check for correct functioning observe:

(1) The general condition of the endoscope, i.e. outside appearance including bending section
(2) The angling and braking system
(3) Optical system
(4) Valve and (if fitted) forceps raiser
(5) Suction and air/water insufflation mechanisms

Cleaning and disinfection

All fibreoptic endoscopes require cleaning and disinfection:

BEFORE USE
AFTER USE

No fibreoptic endoscope should be passed into a patient unless it has been through a satisfactory cleaning and disinfection process. A hospital policy should be worked out with the:

Infection control officer
Microbiologist
Pharmacist

This policy should be planned, implemented and adhered to by all personnel handling the equipment. A suggested policy involves:

(1) Water
(2) Detergent and cleaning brush
(3) Disinfectant
(4) Alcohol

Water

Ordinary tap water can be used for diluting the detergent and for rinsing the endoscope after the use of the detergent and after disinfectant.

Detergent

Washing-up liquid or a bactericidal soapy solution is essential to remove all proteinaceous matter before the instrument is exposed to a disinfecting agent. If this is not done, disinfection will be inadequate and the disinfectant may harden any retained debris, thereby causing blockages.

Disinfectants

A satisfactory disinfectant is vitally important in ensuring the safe practice of gastrointestinal endoscopy. Problems of safety of use for equipment and user

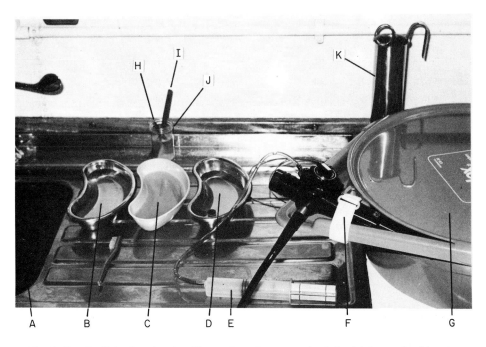

Fig. 2.18 *Facilities for cleaning fibreoptic endoscopes. A, sink with hot and cold water supply and drainage surface; B, receiver for detergent; C, receiver for disinfectant; D, receiver for clean water; E, 50 ml syringe attached to endoscope wash tube; F, controls of endoscope secured by strap; G, container of disinfectant; H, mosquito forceps for handling biopsy forceps; I, tooth brush; J, container for disinfectant; K, container with cheatle forceps for handling accessories in disinfectant container.*

exist with most agents and it is only possible to suggest known products which can be used. Suitable agents are:

2% gluteraldehyde
70% alcohol
Low molecular weight povidone iodine
Povidone iodine
Buffered hypochlorite solutions
Quaternary ammonium concentrates

Sensitivites — gluteraldehyde-based disinfectants are known to cause sensitivites among users. These can be:

Skin rashes
Sinusitis
Conjunctivitis

All personnel using disinfecting agents should:

Wear protective gloves

Avoid splashing

Ensure the ventilation in the endoscopy room is satisfactory

Use as 'closed' a system for the disinfection part of the cleaning cycle as possible e.g. a covered container, cleaning trolley or machine

Personnel experiencing these problems should consult their medical practitioner and establish that the disinfectant is the cause of the symptoms before changing the disinfecting regime.

NB It is not acceptable to stop using a disinfectant altogether in these circumstances as this will give rise to cross infection problems. An alternative agent *must* be introduced.

Alcohol

Before using alcohol of any strength it is important to check with the equipment manufacturer's instructions that it is safe to use on certain parts of a flexible endoscope, and with the pharmacist and Health and Safety Officer that the substance is acceptable for use in the department. 30% alcohol can be used for wiping the outside of the equipment, especially the control body housing as this cleans an area which cannot be cleaned satisfactorily by any other method. It also drys the outside of the endoscope before storage.

Step-by-step cleaning and disinfection of a fibreoptic endoscope at the beginning and the end of an endoscopy list (Fig. 2.18).

---

1. Attach endoscope to light source
2. Attach water-connecting tube from water reservoir
3. Attach suction tube from suction pump
4. Switch on power and *test*:
   (a) Air insufflation by submerging *tip* of endoscope in bowl of water and occluding valve
   (b) Water flow to wash lens by depressing water button
   (c) Suction by occluding suction valve
5. Remove distal hood if present
6. Keeping the controls *dry*, wash the outside of the instrument with a soft disposable cloth
7. Suck detergent through suction/biopsy channel, working forceps raiser up and down (if fitted)
8. Keeping the controls *dry*, remove biopsy valve
9. Pass cleaning brush through suction/biopsy channel, check tip and clean with soft toothbrush *before* withdrawal (Fig. 2.19).
10. Attach wash tube and aspirate detergent through entire length of suction/biopsy channel

continued

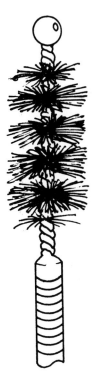

Fig. 2.19   *Endoscope biopsy channel cleaning brush (noted tipped end of brush).*

11. Keeping a finger on the suction button and wiping the instrument free from detergent, remove from detergent
12. Brush the distal tip with a soft toothbrush to remove any residual debris from the air/water nipples and forceps raiser
13. Suck clean water through the suction/biopsy channel
14. Inject weak detergent through the air channel
15. Inject weak detergent through the water channel
16. Remove detergent from air/water channels with clean water
17. Fill water reservoir with disinfectant and blow this through the water channel with the water button
18. Inject disinfectant through the air channel
19. Immerse the shaft of the instrument in disinfectant; fill the suction channel with the agent by attaching a large syringe to the wash tube. Leave the instrument soaking in disinfectant for the time specified by the manufacturers of the disinfectant. Suggested times:

Before and after a list: 20–30 min
Between patients: 5–10 min

continued

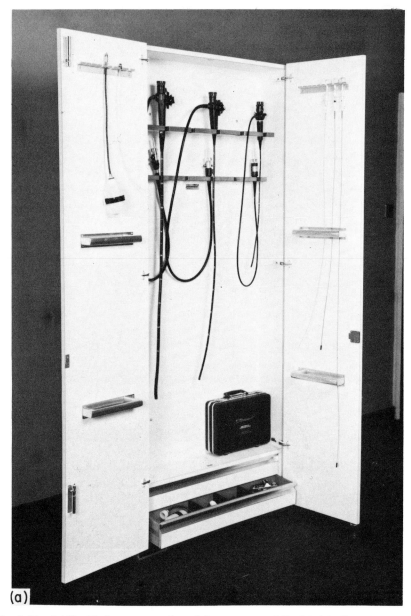

(a)

Fig. 2.20   *(a) KeyMed storage cupboard (by courtesy of KeyMed Ltd).*

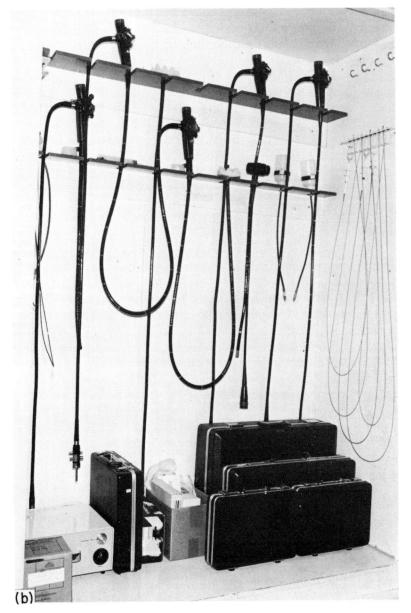

(b)

Fig. 2.20 *(b) Adapted storage cupboard.*

20. At the end of the period of disinfection, remove the endoscope from the container and rinse *all* channels free from disinfectant with clean water
21. Thoroughly *dry* all channels by ensuring all fluid is expelled
22. Wipe dry the outside of the instrument with a swab soaked in 30% alcohol
23. Polish the lens, check the optics and angulation
24. The instrument is now ready for use or storage
25. Fibreoptic endoscopes should be stored vertical in well ventilated security cupboards. Vertical cupboard storage ensures that any remaining moisture drains out and security cupboards are essential to prevent access by unauthorized personnel. Storage cupboards may be purchased complete, or existing space may be adapted (Fig. 2.20).

Cleaning and disinfection procedure between patients

1. On removal of the endoscope from the patient, the air channel should be tested immediately. This prevents any debris travelling up the channel by the Venturi effect and causing a blockage
2. The water button should also be depressed to ascertain that a flow of water is still available. This also ensures that any debris in the water nipple is expelled
3. Any distal hood is removed, and the distal tip cleaned with a soft toothbrush, paying particular attention to a forceps raiser if it is present
4. The shaft of the instrument is washed in detergent with a soft disposable cloth while the suction button is being occluded to aspirate detergent through the suction/biopsy channel
5. Keeping the controls dry, remove biopsy valve and pass the cleaning brush through the channel. Check tip of brush and clean it with a soft toothbrush before withdrawal
6. Clean biopsy valve housing with a 'Q' tip
7. Attach wash tube and aspirate detergent through entire length of suction/biopsy channel
8. Change water bottle for a detergent-filled bottle and flush through water channel
9. Change detergent-filled bottle for a disinfectant-filled bottle and flush through water channel
10. Change disinfectant-filled bottle for a water-filled bottle and flush through water channel
11. Remove from detergent, with a finger on the suction button, and rinse channel and outside of shaft with clean water
12. Remove from clean water, with a finger on the suction button, and

continued

immerse shaft in disinfectant. Attach syringe to wash tube and fill suction/biopsy channel with disinfectant. Allow to soak for maximum length of time available
13. Remove from disinfectant and again rinse channel and outside of instrument in clean water
14. Remove wash tube, dry valve housing with 'Q' tip and fix freshly disinfected valve
15. Ensure all water is aspirated from suction/biopsy channel by occluding the suction button
16. Dry outside of instrument, ensure lenses are clean and the angulation/ breaking system is working and return instrument to trolley ready for the next patient

Light sources

Light sources must be kept clean and dust free. The settings for filters, exposure index, air insufflation and light power should be set according to the user's requirements and the manufacturer's instructions. Spares such as bulbs, air bellows and fuses may be kept in stock for replacement in the smaller light sources. The bigger light sources may require servicing by the equipment distributor and this can be organized on a 'field' service basis or the equipment may have to be returned to the company. When in doubt, consult the company for advice (Fig. 2.21).

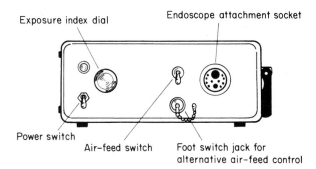

Fig. 2.21 *The front panel of a typical cold-light endoscopy light source.*

Blocked channels

Suction biopsy channel (Fig. 2.22)
(1) Remove valve
(2) Pass brush through to distal tip, clean brush and withdraw

(3) Attach wash tube and suck fluid through the entire length of the instrument.

(4) If the channel is blocked, remove wash tube and replace valve

(5) Attach syringe to suction connection at light source connection and inject water through the cord and out via the suction button

(6) Occlude the suction button and inject water all the way through the endoscope

(7) Should this procedure be unsuccessful the endoscope will require returning to the instrument manufacturer for repair

Air channel (Fig. 2.23(a), (b))

(1) Detach endoscope from light source

(2) Occlude air channel and water inlet

(3) Inject water through air inlet so that it will pass through the entire length of the endoscope

Water channel (Fig. 2.23(c), (d))

(1) Detach endoscope from light source

(2) Press water button fully home and inject water by syringe via the water inlet so that it passes through the entire length of the endoscope

For these purposes a 20 ml or 30 ml syringe is easier to use than a 50 ml or 60 ml syringe. A piece of 'kwill' or fine tubing will be required to attach the syringe to the instrument. If these procedures fail, the endoscope must be returned to the instrument manufacturer for repair.

Hydrogen peroxide

Most blockages are caused by hardened proteinaceous material. Hydrogen peroxide, 10 vols, may be used to help dissolve blockages. It is also advisable to use hydrogen peroxide regularly to ensure channels are kept free from debris and thereby prevent blockages occurring.

Other commercially available agents may be used after consultation with the instrument companies and the pharmacist.

Biopsy valves

A fresh valve must be available for each patient. Valves vary in structure and size to suit different types of endoscopes and in some cases are colour-coded to match the same colour-coding of biopsy forceps.

Cleaning and disinfection

All valves must be dismantled after use, care being taken to clean all separate parts before rinsing and soaking in disinfectant. The parts are dried, lubricated where necessary and reassembled according to the manufacturer's instructions. Some valves may be sterilized by autoclaving after cleaning. Advice should be sought from the manufacturers about methods of sterilization, temperature etc.

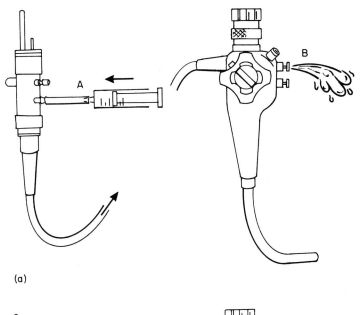

(a)

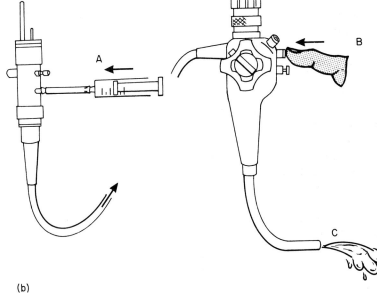

(b)

Fig. 2.22 *(a) Clearing blocked suction/biopsy channel. A, injecting water via suction connection at light guide source connection; B, water flowing out via suction valve. (b) Clearing blocked suction/biopsy channel. A, injecting water via suction connection at light guide source connection; B, depressing suction valve; C, water flowing out via suction inlet.*

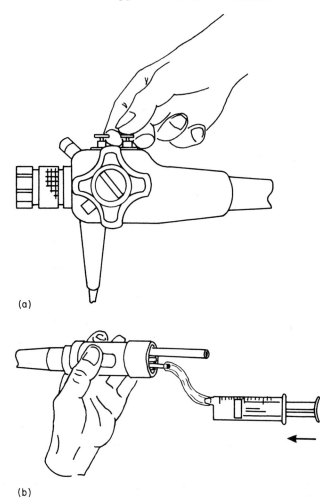

(a)

(b)

Fig. 2.23   Procedure for clearing blocked air/water channel. (a) Close air valve with thumb, (b) close water inlet with thumb and inject water via air inlet.

'Spares' for biopsy valves

Valves must be functioning correctly at all times in order not to damage forceps and other accessories and to prevent leakage of air or aspirated contents over the controls of the endoscope. Depending on the type of valve, it can either be replaced in its entirety (Fig. 2.24(a)), or seals, tapered sleeves and O-rings should all be carefully checked (Fig. 2.24(b)) and replaced when necessary.

Endoscope cleaning machines

Endoscope cleaning machines must always be used according to the instructions of the manufacturers of both the machines and the endoscopes.

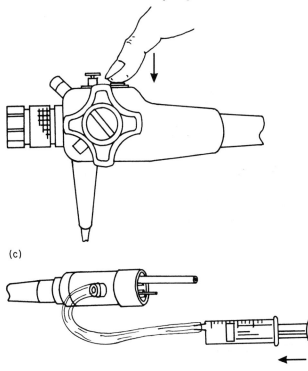

(c)

(d)

Fig. 2.23 *(c) fully depress water button, (d) inject water via water inlet.*

Care must be taken to ensure the safe connection of the machines to the mains supply and any water connections must be secure.

With each machine, it is essential that the following points are noted:

(1) The biopsy channel will require brushing with the cleaning brush and this must be cleaned before withdrawal

(2) The tip of the instrument must be cleaned with a soft toothbrush

(3) Any disinfectant used must be suitable for the endoscope, the machine and the user and have a proven record as a disinfecting agent for infection possibilities in gastroenterology

(4) The endoscope must always be rinsed free of disinfectant

(5) The endoscope must be dried before use or storage

(6) Vertical storage is recommended for all fibreoptic endoscopes

Acmicleanse (AD-1) (Fig. 2.25)

ACM endoscopy has developed its disinfection system to provide for the disinfection of two endoscopes at the same time. The deep top is mounted on a mobile trolley incorporating a circulating pump, disinfectant reservoirs and a large drawer for housing the tubings and connectors.

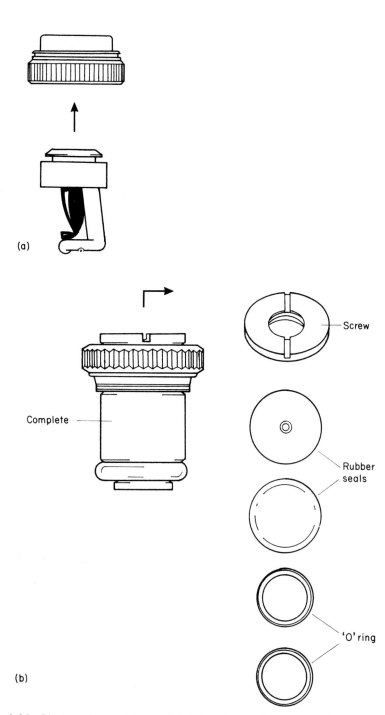

(a)

Screw

Complete

Rubber
seals

'O' ring

(b)

Fig. 2.24 *Biopsy valves. (a) Disposable integral type, (b) rubber seal type.*

The pump is fully automatic being operated by an electronic control. The unit has four variable time cycles: 15 min, 30 min, 45 min and 60 min. It utilizes any standard cleaning/disinfection fluid, a water rinse and a 70% alcohol flush for the quick drying of the air/water and biopsy channels. An easily read digital display indicates the preselected time programme as well as the residual time by means of a reversible counter incorporated in the system. The completion of the cycle is audibly announced. Used tubings and connectors are easily removed and replaced.

Special valve retainers mounted on the top tray ensure that all channels of the endoscopes are held fully open during the circulation of the disinfecting and cleansing fluids. Suitable valve retainers for other manufacturers' instruments are available upon request.

Endocleaner System (Fig. 2.26)

This system, which is manufactured by Georg Pauldrach, is available as a mobile system or as a table model.

By incorporating a precisely controlled low pressure pump with connections to the channels of the endoscope, it ensures circulatory cleaning and disinfection of the channels.

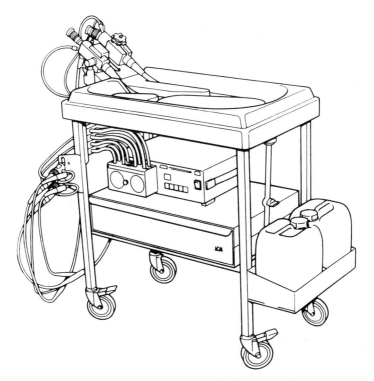

Fig. 2.25 *The Acmicleanse. (Courtesy of ACM Endoscopy Ltd.)*

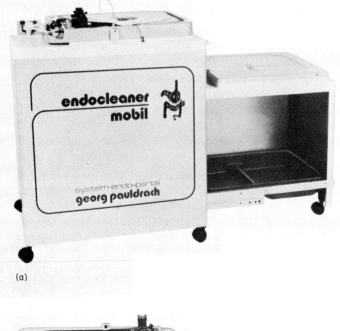

(a)

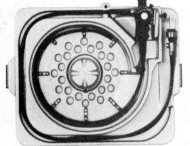

Endocleaner

Control unit
(wall mounted)
table model
also available

Endocleaner cover

Instrument tray

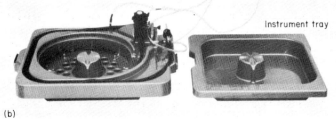

(b)

The system has separate fittings for gastroscopes, colonoscopes and bronchoscopes. It has the ability to clean, disinfect and dry in rapid sequence, so it is of benefit during the endoscopy list.

It only requires access to the mains electrical supply and should be located near a sink. The instrument is rinsed in clean water and cleaned manually immediately after use, then rested in the machine with the connections to both channels attached. The disinfectant is circulated through the channels for the time required, this being controlled by a microprocessor unit. The instrument is then rinsed in clean water and dried prior to use.

KeyMed Fiberscope Disinfectant Irrigator (Fig. 2.27)

This machine cleans and disinfects all channels of Olympus fibrescopes. By irrigating areas which are otherwise inaccessible with detergent/disinfectant, it reduces the risk of bacterial colonization in an endoscope.

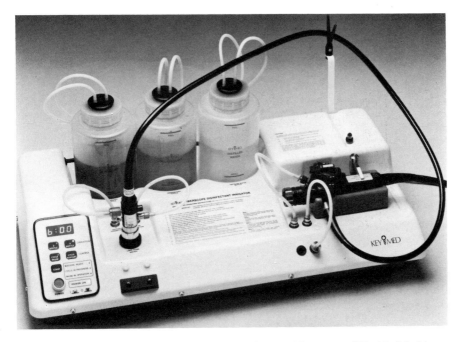

Fig. 2.27 KeyMed Fiberscope Disinfectant Irrigator. (Courtesy of KeyMed Ltd.)

Before use of the irrigator, it is necessary to mechanically clean all accessible parts, including brushing the suction/biopsy channel.

The machine consists of three bottles for detergent, disinfectant and water and a pump, all fitting together into a moulded desk-top mounting. It requires

Fig. 2.26 (a) Endocleaner Mobil, (b) Endocleaner System. (Courtesy of Pyser Ltd.)

a power supply and close access to a sink. Several cradles are supplied which enable connection of the controls of the majority of Olympus endoscopes and throughout the cleaning/disinfecting procedure the distal shaft rests in a bowl in the sink.

After connection, all channels are irrigated by an automatic piston valve system. This system reduces channel blockages to a minimum. There is a choice of a 2-bottle or 3-bottle cycle. A digital read-out and control panel provide simple instructions for cycle timing. The disinfectant hold is unlimited.

The machine does not have a recirculation system, so there are no filters to clean and the machinery is not liable to contamination. All filters and bottles are autoclavable and the machine is portable, quiet and simple to operate and maintain.

Pulstar 1200 Endoscope Processor (Fig. 2.28)

This is a fully automatic portable washer suitable for different types of flexible endoscope. It has two cycles:

(1) Water wash and dry
(2) Water wash, disinfectant delivery and dry

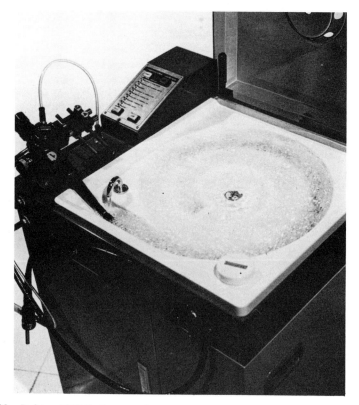

Fig. 2.28   Pulstar 1200 Endoscope Processor (Courtesy of AMSCO Ltd.)

The controls and light guide are clamped into support cradles well clear of the washing area. The flow of water is controlled by a pressure regulator and has two actions:

(1) It is aerated to wash the outside of the shaft of the endoscope in the tray
(2) It flows through the channels by means of valve connections and tubes

Disinfectant can be pumped from the storage tank into the tray to circulate outside the shaft of the instrument and to flow through the channels by the valve connections. Disinfectant is then returned to the storage tank.

Rinsing is by means of aerated water outside the instrument and a flow of water through the channels. Air is blown through the channels after drainage of the water from the tray is completed.

The processor is enclosed and portable. It requires only connection to a mains electricity supply with access to a water tap and drain. The processor has an electronic control system and the fluids are pumped through the channels in a reverse action to the normal flow when the instrument is in use. This method of flow may help ensure improved cleaning of the channels.

Accessories

Biopsy forceps
The structure of forceps gives rise to problems of cleaning and disinfection.

(1) The jaws and, if fitted, the central spike are very small and delicate and after use should be gently cleaned with a soft toothbrush (Fig. 2.29(a)), brushing out any debris or tissue.
(2) The coiled wire structure requires careful cleaning by either gentle scrubbing or by use of an ultrasonic cleaner to ensure that any remaining blood or secretions are removed before the instrument is disinfected. Soaking the wire and distal tip in 10 vols (2.5–3.5%) of hydrogen peroxide may help remove persistent contamination. Disinfection of the forceps is by immersing in the liquid disinfectant of choice, taking care to coil the wire carefully and prevent kinking and to keep the handle clear of the disinfectant
(3) The forceps require thorough rinsing and drying before they are stored either coiled horizontally in drawers or hung on hooks (Fig. 2.30).
(4) Lubrication of the jaws (Fig. 2.29(b)) and the guide-wire (Fig. 2.29(c)) is essential to ensure that the forceps work smoothly when passed through the endoscope
(5) Kinking of the forceps can prevent smooth working of the jaws and may damage the biopsy channel of the endoscope and therefore, damaged forceps should be discarded

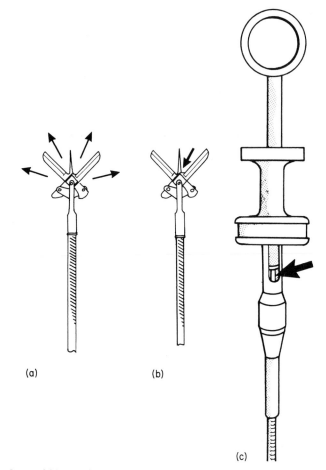

Fig. 2.29   Care of biopsy forceps. (a) Clean jaws with soft toothbrush, (b) lubricate jaws, and (c) lubricate wire in handle.

Cleaning brushes

It is essential to keep cleaning brushes CLEAN with a good bristle tip for adequate cleaning of the endoscope channel.

(1) The tip is scrubbed gently with a soft toothbrush

(2) The coiled wire is scrubbed, care being taken to avoid kinking. The brush can also be cleaned in the ultrasonic cleaner

(3) The brush is disinfected by immersion in liquid disinfectant or by autoclaving

(4) The brush is stored dry either coiled carefully in a drawer or hung on a hook (Fig. 2.30)

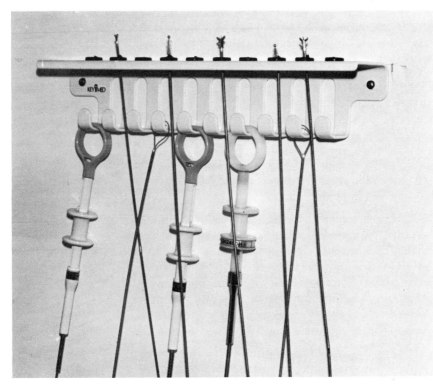

Fig. 2.30   KeyMed accessories storage rack.

Cytology brushes

There are three types of cytology brush:

Unsheathed non-disposable
Sheathed non-disposable
Sheathed disposable

It is important to note that cytology brushes *must* be sterilized by autoclaving if being used more than once, to ensure that all cells are killed.

(1) The brush is removed from sheath if fitted
(2) The tip is scrubbed gently with a soft toothbrush
(3) The coiled wire is cleaned carefully to avoid kinking
(4) If sheathed, the brush is reassembled *with the tip protruding* and immersed in the ultrasonic cleaner
(5) The brush is sent for autoclaving

Disposable brushes can be used in two ways:

(1) The tip is cut off after the sample has been taken and this is sent to the laboratory in a container of cytology fluid

(2) Smears are made with the brush tip on a slide and the brush can either be discarded or reused after the cleaning and disinfection process previously described. It is usually possible to reuse 'disposable' brushes two or three times if the brush is treated with care

Graspers and retrieval instruments

The care of graspers and retrieval instruments is similar to the care of forceps. Care is taken to ensure the moving parts are kept lubricated and in the correct shape in order to function correctly when in use.

Oesophageal dilatation equipment

Each part of the set of equipment used for dilatation of oesophageal strictures must be given individual care.

Guide-wires: require to be cleaned by gentle scrubbing and ultrasonic cleaning of the tip to ensure that residual debris is removed after use. Disinfection may be by liquid disinfectant or by autoclaving. They must be kept smooth and free from kinks to ensure free passage of the guide-wire down the endoscope and free passage of the dilators over the wire. It is important that the flexible tip is firm and smooth at the junction with the wire. If this junction shows signs of weakness or sharpness, the wire must be discarded as it can damage the channel of the endoscope or the mucosa of the oesophagus or stomach.

Olives: require cleaning and disinfection, as for the guide-wires, taking care to replace the olives in the correct order on the tray.

Introducers: the coiled wire design of these make cleaning difficult. After use:

(1) Scrub the outside of the introducer
(2) Attach a syringe (it may be necessary to use polythene tubing to fit the syringe to the introducer and syringe through with detergent to ensure that all blood and debris is removed. It may be necessary to use 10 vols (2.5–3.5%) of hydrogen peroxide to ensure that all blood is removed
(3) Coil in base of ultrasonic cleaner to agitate out remaining debris
(4) Disinfect by liquid disinfectant or sterilize by autoclaving

Flexible tips: after use:

(1) Scrub with a soft toothbrush and check carefully that all residue is removed. Ultrasonic cleaning and syringing with 10 vols hydrogen peroxide ensures that these tips are clean
(2) Disinfect or sterilize as for other parts of the dilating set

NB Check carefully that these tips are in good condition before use, i.e. smooth, firm and with no signs of weakness at the junction (Fig. 2.31), as they can cause damage to the mucosa and even perforation of the stomach wall.

KEEP SPARE GUIDE WIRES AND FLEXIBLE TIPS READILY AVAILABLE!

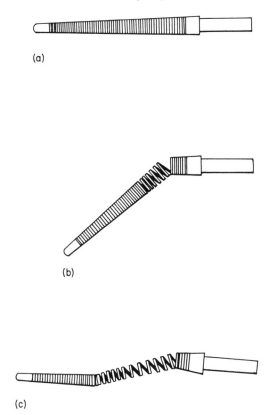

Fig. 2.31 *Flexible tips for Eder–Puestow dilatation system. (a) Correct, (b) dangerous – weakened and bent, (c) dangerous – weakened and stretched.*

Oesophageal intubation equipment

The structure of this equipment is similar to the dilatation equipment and it requires the same care.

(1) The split olives used to maintain the tube in position must be intact, clean and disinfected or sterilized

(2) The locking mechanism should be checked and lubricated

(3) The rammer must be cleaned and disinfected and when required for use, softened in warm water

(4) The rammer cleaning brush must be cleaned and disinfected after use

Mandril system and balloon introducer

(1) After use, wash all parts in detergent

(2) Rinse and disinfect in liquid disinfectant for 20 min

(3) Rinse and dry prior to storage

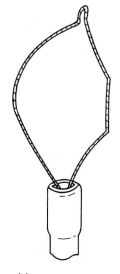

(a)

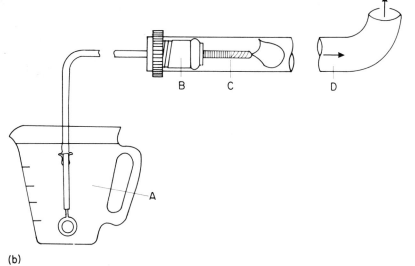

(b)

Fig. 2.32   *(a) Crescent snare for colonoscopic polypectomy. (b) Suction system for cleaning snares; A, jug with detergent; B, biopsy valve; C, accessory, open as for use; D, tubing leading to suction apparatus.*

Cannulae and wash tubes

The correct cannulae must be available for use with the appropriate endoscope. After use:

(1) Syringe with detergent solution to remove any remaining contrast medium

(2) Rinse with clean water

(3) To disinfect: fill lumen with liquid disinfectant and immerse cannulae in container of disinfectant

(4) To sterilize: ascertain correct method and temperatures before submitting any cannulae to autoclaving or steam

Diathermy snares and papillotomes (sphincterotomes) (Fig. 2.32(a))

After use:

(1) Disassemble as far as possible with guidance from manufacturer's literature

(2) Rinse through the tubing with detergent and plain water

(3) Fill lumen of tubing with disinfectant and submerge all parts in liquid disinfectant for recommended period of time

(4) Rinse with clean water followed by 70% alcohol to dry tube lumen

(5) Reassemble, lubricate and test for correct functioning before storage in drawer or cupboard as for biopsy forceps etc.

ALWAYS KEEP SPARE WIRES AND PAPILLOTOMES IN STOCK

NB It is possible to aspirate fluid in a reverse direction through snares etc. by immersing the handle in fluid, passing the accessory through a biopsy valve attached to suction tubing. Accessories may be dried by attaching them to the oxygen supply for a short period and allowing a flow of approximately 6 litres per minute to pass through the tubing (Fig. 2.32(b)).

Sclerotherapy needle (Fig. 2.33)

This instrument is delicate and requires careful handling to prevent:

Damage to the needle tip
Accidental disconnection of catheter tube
Accidental injury to user — the needle tip is sharp!

After use:

(1) On removal from the endoscope, immerse in warm soapy water

(2) Attach syringe and immediately syringe through with warm detergent

(3) Rinse with clean water and empty channel

(4) Fill channel with liquid disinfectant and immerse needle in disinfectant for required length of time

(5) Rinse thoroughly in plain water

(6) Dry inside of channel by syringing through with 70% alcohol

(7) Lubricate proximal end and store instrument in box provided ensuring needle is retracted into the lumen

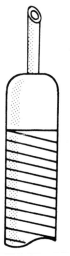

Fig. 2.33 *Sclerotherapy needle showing tip extended.*

CARE OF EQUIPMENT FOR NON-ENDOSCOPIC PROCEDURES

Acid perfusion test equipment

(1) Naso—gastric tubes/Foley catheters: discard after use

(2) Solutions may come from pharmacy manufacturing department in vacolitres: return after use

Gastric function tests

(1) Naso—gastric tubes: discard after use

(2) Suction tubing: if used, discard after each use

(3) Suction pumps: if used, dismantle, clean and disinfect jar; ensure that electrical parts are maintained regularly

Jejunal biopsy capsules

Capsule

Disassemble and clean with detergent after use. A soft toothbrush and cotton buds are useful for cleaning the capsule.

Tubing

Syringe the tubing with detergent and clean water. Fill lumen with disinfectant and immerse in disinfectant for time recommended, along with parts of the capsule. Rinse with clean water, followed by 70% alcohol to dry the lumen of the tube before storage.

CHECK TUBING AT JUNCTION WITH CAPSULE to ensure it is firm. Also check for bite marks at proximal end.

Servicing

To ensure that the blade is sharp and the spring system satisfactory, return capsule to manufacturer for regular servicing.

Breath test equipment

(1) Disassemble tube, needle and syringe vial
(2) Discard drying agent
(3) Wash equipment in detergent and rinse in plain water
(4) Soak parts in disinfectant
(5) Rinse in clean water, dry and store ready for use

If using a proprietary machine, follow manufacturer's instructions.

Meditech steerable catheter jejunal biopsy system

Handle

Disconnect from catheter, wipe with alcohol swab. Check screws are fitted and lubricate if necessary.

Steerable Catheter

(1) Check all wires are intact and of the correct tension
(2) Remove capsule tip and clean
(3) Remove blade with care and clean with brush in detergent
(4) Immerse blade and capsule tip in disinfectant
(5) Syringe catheter with detergent and clean water
(6) Fill lumen with disinfectant and immerse up to control end
(7) Rinse with clean water
(8) Dry lumen with 70% alcohol
(9) Replace blade and capsule
(10) Store in box provided

Care of the laparoscope

Thorough cleaning and sterilization of the laparoscope and its accessories before and after use is essential.

Before use

(1) All parts should be inspected and in perfect working order before cleaning

(a) Laparoscope. The lenses must be clear. Polish with lens wax if necessary. The seal must fit well. Replace when worn

(b) Light carrier. Check that there are no perforations

(c) Trocar and cannula. The seal must fit well. Replace when worn. Trumpet valve – disassemble, lubricate with silicone and then reassemble

(d) Teaching attachment. Check this and clean the lens with wax

(2) Wash the parts described above in detergent solution. Brush through the biopsy channel of the laparoscope with a cleaning brush and gently brush the lens using a soft toothbrush

(3) Immerse completely in 2% gluteraldehyde for at least 3 hours

(4) After this time all parts must be thoroughly rinsed in sterile water before use

After use

(1) All equipment must be thoroughly washed in detergent solution

(a) Laparoscope. Brush through the biopsy channel with a cleaning brush. Remove the eye-piece and using a toothbrush, clean the proximal and distal lens. Remove and wash the seal

(b) Light carrier. Wash well

(c) Trocar and cannula. Wash the trocar. Dismantle the cannula and brush through. Clean all parts with a soft toothbrush

(d) Teaching attachment. Wash well and brush lens with a soft toothbrush.

(2) All above items are then disinfected in gluteraldehyde for at least 20 min

(3) Items which must be sterilised by steam sterilization are:

Menghini needle
Verres needle
Tactile probe
Insufflation tubing
Insertion tubes for pre-heater

They should be cleaned in detergent, rinsed and dried immediately after use prior to sterilization. Any moving parts require lubrication *before sterilization.*

After disinfection (items (a)–(d))

(1) Rinse well in water and dry with absorbent towels and gauze

(2) The laparoscope and teaching attachment should be wiped over with 70% alcohol and dried with gauze. The lenses should be cleaned and polished using lens wax

(3) The cannula trumpet valve should be lubricated with silicone and re-assembled

(4) Correct storage and maintenance of all equipment is essential

THE ENDOSCOPY ROOM

All endoscopic investigations and therapeutic procedures are best carried out in a purpose-designed room. The room requires to contain:

Work surfaces
Sink with drainer surface
Storage space for drugs, needles, syringes etc.
An endoscopy trolley
Cleaning and disinfection facilities for endoscopes and accessories
Wash basin for staff use
Writing surface, telephone, radiograph viewing boxes
Resuscitation equipment

There must be sufficient remaining floor space to accommodate the patient trolley plus endoscopist and his assisting staff. Endoscopy may be carried out on a fixed table and if this is so there will be a requirement for space for the patient to be wheeled in on a separate trolley and transferred across. Some endoscopy rooms may be equipped with an image intensifier and provision for radiological screening. In a teaching environment, CCTV may be provided and this will also require space.

When endoscopic procedures require radiology facilities, equipment will need to be transferred to the Radiology department. Care must be taken to ensure that the equipment is not damaged in transit. Adaption of the existing layout of the Radiology room is necessary to ensure a safe and satisfactory procedure. It is essential that the same standard of patient and equipment care is maintained on these occasions as in the purpose-designed room.

Hints on furnishings for the endoscopy room

It is possible to obtain professional help in planning accommodation for use as an endoscopy room or Gastroenterology department. Having established the service to be provided and planned for future changes and expansion, it is possible to decide on requirements for alterations to existing space, furnishings and equipment.

Work surfaces

The maximum amount of work surfaces should be utilized in the room and they should be of a type which can be wiped clean easily. It is preferable that they have a raised edge to ensure expensive equipment does not slip to the floor.

Sinks

Sinks require to have at least one drainer surface. Mixer taps are useful but not essential. A separate handbasin should be fitted for staff hand washing.

Storage space

Storage space is important to keep equipment safe. Cupboards and drawers require to be of smooth material and as spacious as possible. If endoscopes are to be stored in the room, security cupboards can be fitted to the wall. More spacious cupboards can be adapted from previous ward or department store cupboards.

An endoscopy trolley

As previously described an endoscopy trolley is provided and equipped with such items as syringes, lubricant, cameras etc. Depending on the layout it may be possible to utilize fitted accommodation for the same purpose.

Cleaning and disinfection equipment

This will depend on the amount of space available and the system chosen. Endoscopes can be cleaned by:

(1) A machine specially designed to wash, disinfect and dry the equipment
(2) A specially designed cleaning and disinfection trolley
(3) A system adapted to suit the layout of the room

Drug cupboards

These should be fitted to comply with hospital drug regulation.

Refrigerator

A drug refrigerator may be required for the storage of some drugs in use.

Resuscitation equipment

Full resuscitation facilities are essential and should comply with hospital requirements. Oxygen, either piped or cylinder, should be readily available.

Suction equipment

Suction equipment is required for the patient and the endoscope, and this can either be piped or free standing suction.

Preparing the room for use

(1) Clean work surfaces and the endoscopy trolley
(2) Lay up trolley with endoscope and accessories to be used
(3) Test and disinfect endoscope
(4) Draw up drugs required
(5) Check resuscitation equipment, oxygen and patient suction
(6) If preferred, the equipment to be used may be covered until the patient is sedated

(7) Prepare essential documentation and ensure that the notes and radiographs of the patient are in the room

(8) Check that the room temperature, the lighting and ventilation are satisfactory

(9) Keep the room door closed during the procedure

(10) Have ready detergent, disinfectant and other cleaning requirements to allow for a quick turn round between patients

3

THE UPPER GASTROINTESTINAL TRACT

THE OESOPHAGUS

Anatomy

The oesophagus is a muscular tube which connects the mouth to the stomach. It starts in the neck at the lower part of the pharynx where it lies behind the trachea and in front of the cervical vertebrae. Throughout the thorax the oesophagus remains applied to the vertebral column posteriorly, whilst anteriorly, it is related to the trachea in its upper portion and then to the heart. It passes out of the chest at the diaphragmatic orifice where it joins the stomach at the gastro—oesophageal junction (cardia). The oesophagus has sphincter muscles at its upper end (cricopharyngeal) and its lower end (cardiac). These relax during the act of swallowing.

Throughout most of its length the oesophagus is lined by squamous epithelium. Just above the stomach, at the gastro—oesophageal junction, the mucosa becomes columnar in character. The squamocolumnar junction is at a variable distance from the incisor teeth but most commonly occurs at approximately the level of the diaphragm, namely 38—45 cm from the teeth. The level of mucosal change may be referred to as the 'Z' line or dentate line.

Physiology

The most important role of the oesophagus is to transfer food from the mouth to the stomach. This is achieved by the act of swallowing. Once food has passed from the mouth into the oesophagus by the action of the mouth and pharyngeal muscles, the onward movement of the food bolus is an involuntary act. Sequential contractions and relaxation of the circular muscles in the wall of the oesophagus propel the food down the oesophagus and into the stomach in approximately twenty seconds. The mechanism whereby the circular muscles behind a bolus of food contract whilst those directly in front relax, thus forcing the food onwards down the oesophagus, is called 'peristalsis'.

Pathology

Hiatus hernia and reflux oesophagitis

The most common disorder of the oesophagus is reflux oesophagitis. Here the mechanisms which maintain acid gastric contents within the stomach have become incompetent and reflux of gastric contents occurs frequently, leading to inflammation of the lower portion of the oesophagus. The patient complains of a burning sensation behind the breast bone especially in recumbency or upon stooping. Sometimes the reflux is so severe as to cause the mouth to fill with acid. Contributory factors to the production of reflux are:

Obesity
Pregnancy
Stooping
Lying flat
Smoking
Excessive alcohol consumption
Large meals
Hiatus hernia
Gallstones

A hiatus hernia is present when the diaphragmatic orifice through which the oesophagus passes is too large. Under these circumstances, a 'knuckle' of stomach passes through the diaphragm in an upward direction into the chest. As a result, the lower oesophageal sphincter mechanism is distorted and inadequate. Symptoms of reflux as described above are the cardinal symptoms of a hiatus hernia, but may be associated with excessive flatulence and difficulty with swallowing (dysphagia). Rarely, ulceration may occur within the herniated stomach or in the oesophagus just above it. Bleeding may occur and anaemia may result. More seriously in the long term, repeated ulceration of the oesophagus may result in a stricture at its lower end.

Oesophageal carcinoma

At its lower end, the oesophagus may be the site of an adenocarcinoma. This may occur within the oesophagus itself due to the presence of ectopic columnar mucosa or as a result of encroachment upwards from a gastric primary growth. More commonly, the oesophagus is the site of a squamous-celled carcinoma which occurs within the territory of the squamous oesophageal lining previously described.

Disordered motility

Sometimes the regular muscular contraction within the oesophagus becomes

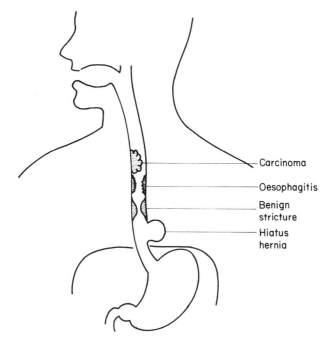

Fig. 3.1 Common disorders of the oesophagus.

deranged and normal swallowing cannot occur. Most commonly, such oesophageal spasms are related to the presence of other primary conditions of the
oesophagus such as reflux oesophagitis or the presence of a hiatus hernia.
Rarely, the condition is due to an infiltration into the oesophageal wall in conditions such as systemic scleroderma or amyloidosis. Occasionally, the
abnormal muscular contractions occur when no obvious cause can be found.

In achalasia of the cardia, the normal neuromuscular structures are absent or
damaged in a short segment of the oesophagus just above the stomach. The
resultant dysphagia and hold-up in the oesophagus may be relieved by surgery.
Techniques have been developed whereby pneumatic dilatation of the oesophagus may achieve equally good results.

STOMACH AND DUODENUM

Anatomy (Fig. 3.2)

The stomach is a saccular reservoir lying in the left upper quadrant of the
abdomen. Here, digestive processes are initiated since food is retained in this
area for 2–4 hours after swallowing. The stomach starts at the cardia, which is
where the oesophagus finishes, and the J-shaped organ ends at a firm muscular
ring called the pylorus through which partially digested foodstuffs pass into the

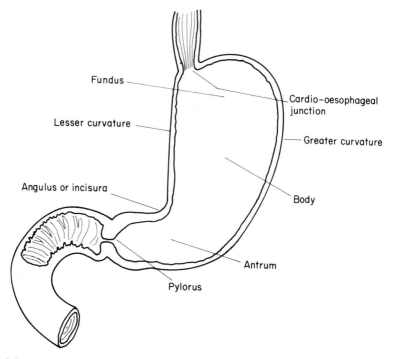

Fig. 3.2   *Anatomy of the stomach.*

duodenum. The stomach lies in close relationship to the diaphragm above and the coils of small intestine beneath. Posteriorly, the 'stomach-bed' is formed in part by the spleen, left kidney, pancreas and great vessels. Anteriorly, the stomach lies in close relationship to the anterior abdominal wall. Exit from the stomach via the pylorus leads directly into the duodenum which is a tubular structure about 30 cm long. It is roughly 'C' shaped and cradles the head of the pancreas within it. It is divided into the first part or bulb, the second part or descending duodenum, and the third and fourth parts. Beyond the fourth part the duodenum leads directly into the small intestine.

Within the stomach, certain landmarks are important to the endoscopist. On entering the stomach from the oesophagus at the cardia, the endoscopist first identifies the prominent longitudinal folds of the greater curvature of the stomach, which are situated on the patient's left. These start in the capacious fundus of the stomach and run down into the main body of the stomach. Opposite lies the rather featureless lesser curve, which ends distally at a crescent-shaped mucosal fold called the incisura or angulus. The anterior gastric wall lies between these two areas to the front, whilst the posterior aspect of the stomach lies between the greater and lesser curves posteriorly. If the endoscopist then follows the folds of the greater curvature downwards, the saccular gastric antrum is entered. This starts at the level of the incisura on the lesser curve. The antrum leads directly to the pylorus which can usually be seen as a small dark hole intermittently screened by waves of peristaltic contractions. Endoscopically, the duodenum differs in appearance from the body of the stomach. The bulb is seen as a saccular structure just beyond the pylorus with a prominent mucosal fold, the superior duodenal fold, separating it from the second part. On the medial wall of the second part of the duodenum, the ampulla of Vater can be seen. Here the pancreatic and common bile ducts emerge into the duodenum. Sometimes an additional or accessory ampulla may be seen. Below this level, the duodenum is a long tube with prominent concentric mucosal folds, the valvulae conniventes.

Structurally, the wall of the stomach comprises four layers:

The mucous membrane, the cells of which produce gastric juice consisting of the digestive enzyme pepsin, hydrochloric acid and mucus

The submucosal layer which forms a structural skeleton and contains supportive tissues and blood vessels

A muscular layer, consisting of circular, longitudinal and oblique muscle layers. At the cardia and the pylorus, the circular muscle layers are more dense and form sphincters

The outer layer or serosa which forms part of the peritoneal covering

The wall of the duodenum is of similar construction.

Physiology

The stomach is a large reservoir for food received from the oesophagus and it is the area where the digestive process is initiated. As food enters the stomach, the organ relaxes to accommodate it and retains the whole meal in the stomach during the gastric stage of digestion. Here, the food is churned and thoroughly mixed with gastric juice prior to onward delivery into the duodenum. Studies have shown that mixing is controlled by a gastric pacemaker situated near the cardia which initiates gastric contractions at the rate of three per minute.

Gastric contents enter the duodenum via the pylorus under the influence of peristaltic contractions of the gastric antrum at the same rate. This mechanism is known as the antral pump and is produced by co-ordinated contractions in the antrum, pylorus and first part of the duodenum. Posture and gravity have little effect on gastric emptying which occurs progressively over a 2–4 hour period, liquids being ejected more rapidly than solids. The vagus nerve and its distribution, is important in controlling gastric emptying. For example, after a truncal vagotomy gastric stasis is commonplace, but if the nerve supply to the antrum is preserved, in a highly selective vagotomy, gastric retention does not occur.

Several factors control the rate of gastric emptying. These are:

The constituents of the meal
The osmolarity of the meal

The pH of the meal
Inhibitory impulses from the wall of the duodenum and upper jejunum

It seems probable that this control is effected through osmoreceptors and pH receptors. In consequence, hyperosmolar substances may slow the rate of gastric emptying. Once into the duodenum, fat and acid contents of a meal stimulate the release of further hormones which initiate the next acts of digestion. These important hormones are secretin, cholecystokinin, motilin and vasoinhibitory polypeptide (VIP). Although the exact inter-relationship of these hormones is not entirely clear in normal gastric control, the area is one of great importance because duodenal reflux of bile and duodenal contents may play an important role in the production of gastric ulcer and reflux oesophagitis. In uncomplicated duodenal ulcer, gastric emptying is usually more rapid whereas it is delayed in patients with antral gastric ulcers and gastric cancer. Delayed gastric emptying may also be observed in uraemia, migraine and autonomic neuropathy such as that seen in diabetes mellitus.

Secretion

Even before food arrives in the stomach, nervous mechanisms will have initiated gastric secretion. Factors which will have initiated secretion via vagus nerve routes are as follows:

Conditional meal times
Hypoglycaemia
The smell, taste and chewing of food
Emotional states

These factors all act via the brain at hypothalamic level and subsequently via the sympathetic and parasympathetic nerve pathways. Sympathetic stimulation initiates gastric secretion by increasing gastric blood flow, whilst parasympathetic stimulation effects gastric secretion via vagal influence on gastric parietal cells. Antral vagal stimulation also promotes gastrin release from the G cells of this area. Gastrin passes into the circulation where it stimulates both acid and pepsinogen secretion. As food enters the stomach, the gastric phase of secretion is initiated by distension. Secretion is stimulated both locally and by longer vagal reflex arcs. Antral stimulation, by distension and protein content of the meal, stimulates further gastrin release.

Acid secretion

Acid secretion results from the interaction of long tract vagal stimulation from the base of the brain and local stimulation through reflex arcs. Although histamine has been suggested as the final common stimulator of parietal cells acting at the histamine H_2 receptor site, the exact relationship between acetylcholine, histamine and gastrin remains to be clarified.

Pepsin secretion

Pepsin secretion results from the release of pepsinogen granules which have been stored in the parietal or chief cells of the gastric fundus. Once discharged, the pepsinogen granules are activated to pepsin by both gastric acid and subsequently by pepsin itself. Pepsin secretion parallels that of gastric acid, and can be reduced by vagotomy, the administration of atropine and H_2 receptor antagonists, as well as by gastric mucosal atrophy.

Intrinsic factor secretion

Instrinsic factor is secreted by the parietal cells of the healthy gastric body and its production parallels gastric acid secretion. Production is stimulated by insulin, histamine or gastrin. Intrinsic factor is essential for binding vitamin B_{12} for subsequent absorption in the terminal ileum. Patients with gastric mucosal atrophy or previous gastric surgery, may have a deficiency of intrinsic factor leading to vitamin B_{12} deficiency.

Gastrin

Gastrin, a polypeptide hormone, was isolated in 1964 and is probably the best understood hormone of the gastrointestinal tract because of its well-studied stimulatory effect in gastric acid secretion. Several forms of gastrin exist and dependent upon the number of component amino acids, they are known as 'big gastrin', 'big, big gastrin' and 'mini-gastrin'. Gastrin is found most commonly in granules of cytoplasm of big G cells situated in the gastric antrum, but they may also be identified in the islets of Langerhan's in the pancreas, and in the tumour cells of a gastrinoma which most commonly occurs in the pancreas.

Secretin

Secretin is a hormone which has a chain of 27 amino acids. It is secreted by cells in the duodenal mucosa when acid gastric contents are released from the stomach. Secretin has an important role in the stimulation of the pancreas to produce a solution rich in bicarbonate which neutralizes acid gastric contents.

Inhibition of gastrin

Gastric secretion normally continues for one to two hours following ingestion of a meal before a number of inhibitory mechanisms come into action. Once the acidity of gastric contents is below pH 2.5, antral gastrin release is inhibited. Once protein and fat enter into the duodenum, the secretion of cholecystokinin and pancreozymin acts to reduce acid gastric secretion and gastric motility whilst initiating pancreatic secretion, gall bladder contraction and hepatic secretion. The overall effect of these actions is to produce a flow of alkaline bile and pancreatic juice which neutralizes the acid meal within the lumen of the duodenum and so begin the intestinal phase of digestion.

Mucosal resistance to injury

The gastric mucosa is resistant to damage by its own secretions. Auto digestion is prevented by the presence of gastric mucus and the epithelial barrier. Large quantities of mucus are produced by the gastric mucosa if irritant food or drink are ingested. The viscosity of mucus changes with pH. It does not buffer acid but probably absorbs pepsin. In addition to this effect, the epithelial lining cells of the gastric mucosa are able to regenerate in 36–48 hours. The cellular lining is liable to damage by salicylates, bile salts and alcohol. Once damage occurs, the permeability of the epithelial lining is increased allowing back-diffusion of hydrogen ions from the gastric contents, thus initiating damage to the underlying tissues.

Pathology (Fig. 3.3)

Peptic ulcer

The term 'peptic' ulcer refers to an ulcer in the lower oesophagus, stomach, duodenum, jejunum after gastric surgery or, rarely, in the ileum in a Meckel's diverticulum. Ulcers in the stomach or duodenum may be acute or chronic and may penetrate to the muscular layers. Acute ulcers heal without fibrosis.

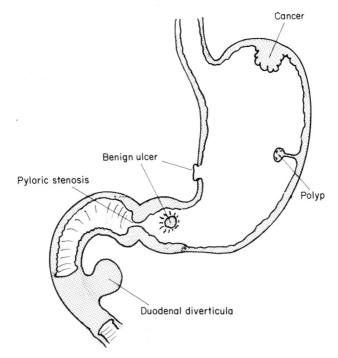

Fig. 3.3   *Important disorders of the stomach and duodenum.*

Although the incidence of peptic ulceration is decreasing in Western countries, it still affects approximately 10% of all adult males. The male to female ratio varies from 4:1 to 2:1 in different communities, whilst that for gastric ulcer is 2:1 or even less. Peptic ulceration is becoming progesssively more common in developing countries. The aetiology of peptic ulceration is multifactorial.

Heredity

Patients with peptic ulcer often have a family history of the disease; this is especially so when duodenal ulcers affect young people. However, gastric and duodenal ulcers are inherited as separate disorders. The relatives of families with gastric ulcers have three times the expected number of duodenal ulcers, whilst duodenal ulcers occur within the family with the same frequency as within the general population.

The mucosal barrier

The immediate cause of peptic ulceration is the digestion of the mucosa by acid and pepsin of gastric juice, but the sequence of events is unclear. Destructive forces include hydrochloric acid and pepsin produced by the stomach. In addition, psychogenic factors, reflux of duodenal contents including bile and pancreatic juice, nicotine, analgesics and anti-inflammatory drugs may also have an adverse effect on the gastric mucosal barrier. It is probable that an ulcer develops when these attacking factors outweigh the defensive factors (Fig. 3.4).

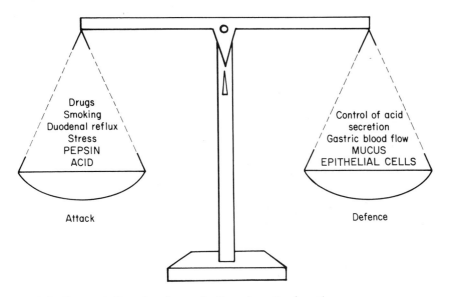

Fig. 3.4   *Factors influencing the production of peptic ulceration.*

Peptic ulcer in special circumstances

Acute and stress ulcers

Many of the factors described above also contribute to the development of acute ulcers. Aspirin and non-steroidal anti-inflammatory analgesics are especially important but acute peptic ulcers may develop after head injury, burns, severe sepsis, surgery or trauma. Gastric hypersecretion is the usual cause of acute ulcers after head injury whilst reflux of duodenal contents or mucosal ischaemia may be responsible factors after burns, shock or hypotension.

Post-bulbar ulcer

Although the commonest site of peptic ulceration within the duodenum lies in the duodenal bulb or cap, ulcers may occasionally occur in the post-bulbar region. This lies just into the second part of the duodenum and is a difficult area to visualize radiologically. Occasionally, endoscopic inspection of the area in patients who have radiologically negative dyspepsia will provide the diagnosis. This possibility justifies endoscopic inspection of the second part of the duodenum in all routine upper gastrointestinal endoscopy.

Benign gastric ulcer

Benign gastric ulcer is nearly always a solitary lesion and 90% are situated on the lesser curve of the stomach within the antrum or at the junction between body and antral mucosa. Acute ulcers or erosions are frequently multiple and are much more widely distributed. The most important distinction to be made between duodenal and gastric ulcers is that the latter may be malignant. It is the clinician's responsibility to exclude malignancy in gastric ulceration.

Gastritis

The term gastritis signifies an acute or chronic inflammation of the stomach. It is a term which has been loosely applied to the appearance of reddening of the gastric mucosa identified endoscopically. There is, however, a poor relationship between the endoscopic appearances and histological evidence of true inflammation. Indeed, it is rare to find histological specimens taken from a normal stomach which are completely free from any signs of inflammation. In this sense, gastritis is almost an invariable finding in adults. Gross departures from this situation do, however, occur. Acute gastritis is most commonly caused by the ingestion of aspirin, antirheumatic drugs and alcohol. It may also be caused by the regurgitation of bile into the stomach especially after gastric surgery. Despite the findings of a reddened mucosa and histological evidence of inflammation, the condition is probably asymptomatic.

In chronic gastritis, there is a progressive reduction of the specialized glands of the body of the stomach and lymphocytic infiltration of the mucosa. Atrophic gastritis results in a reduction of the thickness of the mucosa although round cell infiltration is slight. Chronic gastritis is common in gastric ulcer, gastric cancer and after gastric surgery. Pernicious anaemia is invariably accompanied by chronic gastritis and under these circumstances, circulating antibodies to parietal cells and intrinsic factor are frequently found. Chronic gastritis is certainly asymptomatic and its importance lies in association with the disorders noted above. The diagnosis can only be confirmed by gastric biopsy.

Tumours of the stomach

Carcinoma of the stomach

Carcinoma of the stomach is one of the most common malignant tumours of the gastrointestinal tract, although its incidence varies in different parts of the world. These variations in incidence have been attributed to environmental factors such as trace elements in the water or to differences in method of food preparation. The highest incidence of gastric ulcer worldwide occurs in Japan. In addition to these environmental factors, patients with pernicious anaemia and those who have undergone previous gastric surgery have an increased risk of developing gastric cancer.

Almost 70% of all gastric cancers occur at the pylorus or in the antrum. Symptoms of obstruction to the gastric outlet are common. Lesions of the body of the stomach most commonly involve the greater curvature and produce a fungating ulcerated mass. Much less common is a diffuse infiltrating carcinoma spreading throughout the body of the stomach and producing the so-called leather-bottle stomach. In the early stages, when the carcinoma is confined to the mucosa, the lesion may be particularly difficult to detect since it may be represented only by a depressed area, distortion of the mucosal folds or by shallow irregular ulceration. Endoscopy is an important diagnostic aid at this early stage when the tumour is potentially curable by resection. Gastric cancer may present as a malignant ulcer. Most authorities believe that chronic peptic ulcer of the stomach rarely becomes malignant and that malignant ulcers, however long they have been present, have always been malignant. The most important role of the clinician is to decide whether a chronic gastric ulcer is benign or malignant with all measures available to him since the diagnosis of the lesion at an early stage may improve prognosis.

In general, prognosis is very poor and the only means currently available by which it can be improved, is by detection of the early lesion. This requires a vigorous approach to the problem of dyspepsia in the middle-aged, including careful radiological and endoscopic examination with critical follow-up of doubtful abnormalities.

Benign tumours of the stomach

Tiny mucosal polyps are a frequent finding at endoscopy. Their presence is of questionable significance and they probably represent mucosal regeneration after an injury such as acute gastritis. It is however, important to exclude early malignant change and on this basis, endoscopic biopsies are essential.

Rarely, a solitary polypoid lesion with a friable haemorrhagic head, may occur in the stomach. The importance of this lesion is its proneness to cause recurrent gastrointestinal bleeding and the ease with which it may be removed endoscopically with diathermy.

A leiomyoma of the stomach may present as a tumour mass with an ulcerated surface. Although benign, these rare tumours have a tendency to become malignant at a later stage and surgery is indicated for their removal.

Upper gastrointestinal haemorrhage

Haemorrhage from the upper gastrointestinal tract presenting as haematemesis or melaena is a common cause for admission to hospital. Bleeding of this nature may be responsible for up to 1% of acute medical admissions. The common causes of bleeding are:

Gastric and duodenal ulcers
Gastric erosions
Oesophageal varices
Lacerations at the cardia due to vomiting (Mallory–Weiss syndrome)

Less frequent causes of gastrointestinal haemorrhage are:

Cancer of the stomach and other tumours such as polyps or leiomyomas
Oesophagitis
Acute stress ulcers and bleeding disorders
Vascular abnormalities

In recent years it has become apparent that endoscopy is the most valuable investigation in elucidating the source of gastrointestinal haemorrhage. Despite this, earlier more accurate diagnosis has not been shown to significantly alter the prognosis in the condition. Mortality may reach 30% in elderly and shocked patients. Aspects of this subject are dealt with in Chapter 8.

Previous gastric surgery

Whilst most operations upon the stomach are highly successful, a small number of patients have recurrent symptoms at a variable time after their gastric surgery. These symptoms may be due to bile reflux, which may cause gastritis or reflux oesophagitis, or to the presence of an ulcer occurring at the anastomotic site. Flatulence and distension are common symptoms. Endoscopy is a valuable investigation under these circumstances since radiology is less reliable as a result of the previous gastric surgery. In addition, there is an increased risk of gastric malignancy at a late stage in previous gastrectomy and endoscopy should be undertaken in symptomatic patients to clarify these points.

Zollinger–Ellison syndrome

The rare condition of Zollinger–Ellison syndrome is characterized by recurrent severe gastric and duodenal ulceration. Diarrhoea may be an accompaniment. The condition is caused by overproduction of the hormone gastrin, most commonly by a tumour situated in the pancreas. Gastric acid output studies, serum gastrin level estimations and endoscopy are valuable diagnostic aids. In patients with the Zollinger–Ellison syndrome, serum gastrin levels rise after injection of secretion. This forms the basis of the secretin-infusion test which may be useful in sorting out patients with equivocal results.

Duodenal polyps

Polyps may occur in the first and second part of the duodenum. They are most commonly benign and are produced by regeneration of mucosa after peptic ulceration. Malignant lesions of the duodenum are rare.

Ampullary carcinoma

Carcinoma of the ampulla of Vater may present with jaundice as a result of obstruction to bile outflow by the malignant lesion of the ampulla. Endoscopic inspection of the second part of the duodenum can readily establish the diagnosis.

Mucosal lesions of the duodenum

The mucosal lesion of coeliac disease which is most commonly found in the jejunum, also affects the duodenal mucosa. Sometimes, the mosaic pattern of the atrophic mucosa of the condition may be seen on routine endoscopic inspection. Alternatively, mucosal abnormalities may be detected by spraying a dye such as methylene blue onto the surface. Endoscopic biopsies of abnormal mucosa under these circumstances may be just as useful in confirming the diagnosis of coeliac disease as the more formal approaches to jejunal biopsy using biopsy capsules.

INVESTIGATIONS AND THERAPEUTIC PROCEDURES

Barium swallow and meal

The commonest technique used to investigate the presence of upper gastrointestinal disorders is the barium swallow and meal. The patient is asked to swallow mouthfuls of a radio-opaque suspension of barium which outlines the oesophagus and stomach. In the oesophagus, the technique is excellent for detecting hiatus hernia, cancer and disturbed motility. Reflux oesophagitis, oesophageal varices and early cancer can sometimes be missed by this technique. In the stomach and duodenum, peptic ulcer and malignant lesions can

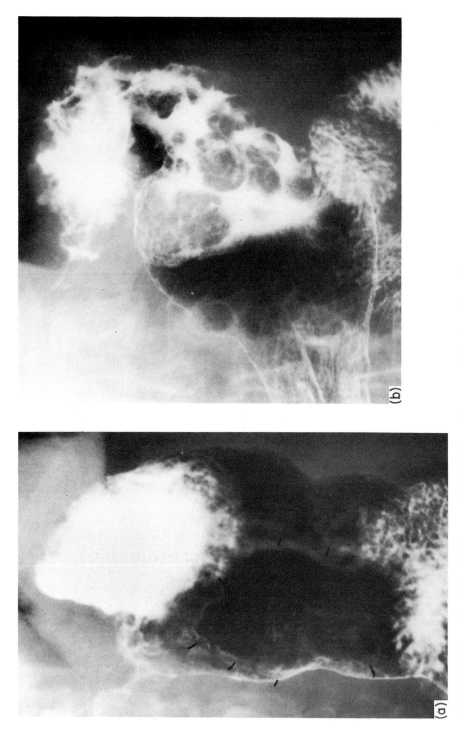

Fig. 3.5 Lesions detected by barium meal. (a) 'Flat' gastric cancer, (b) polypoid gastric cancer.

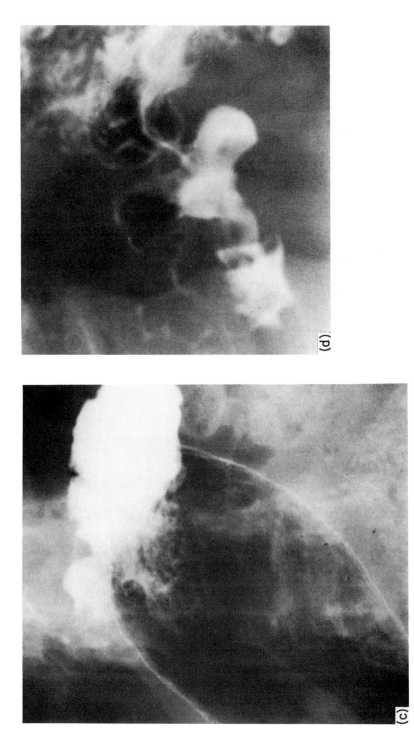

Fig. 3.5 (c) Hiatus hernia, and (d) duodenal ulcer.

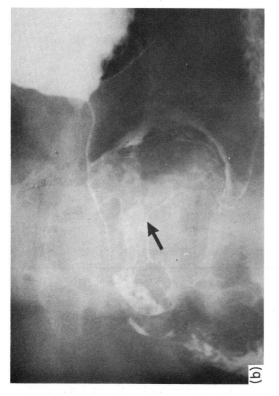

(b)

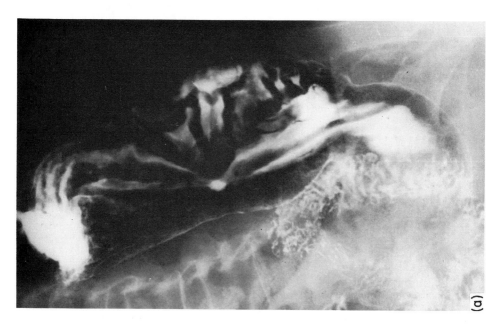

(a)

Fig. 3.6 Double-contrast barium meal showing (a) benign gastric ulcer with radiating mucosal folds and (b) antral carcinoma.

usually be detected radiologically, especially if a double contrast technique is used. Even with the double contrast technique, lesions can sometimes be missed, and radiology and upper gastrointestinal endoscopy should be used jointly to establish a diagnosis (Figs 3.5 and 3.6).

Upper gastrointestinal endoscopy

Fibreoptic inspection of the upper gastrointestinal tract is a technique which provides good visualization of the mucosal lining of the oesophagus, stomach and duodenum with a chance to observe pathological changes, peristaltic movements of the respective parts and an opportunity to take biopsies or perform therapeutic procedures down the endoscope. The patient needs very little pre-operative preparation and is usually requested to starve for a minimum of four hours prior to the procedure during ideal circumstances. This allows gastric emptying, thus permitting better visualization and reducing the risk of regurgitation of gastric contents and aspiration of them into the respiratory tract. An endoscopic service will run more smoothly if the administrative back-up described elsewhere in this book can be established.

Upper gastrointestinal endoscopy is a better investigation than the barium swallow and meal in certain circumstances (Tables 3.1 and 3.2). In particular, where biopsies of a lesion are required or when the site of upper gastrointestinal haemorrhage is in question, then endoscopy is the preferred investigation. In addition, various therapeutic procedures such as dilatation of oesophageal strictures or sclerotherapy of oesophageal varices can only be performed endoscopically.

The technique of endoscopy varies but usually the patient's throat will be anaesthetized with local anaesthetic and a small dose of intravenous sedation administered. It is not necessary to render the patient totally unconscious and it is beneficial to the endoscopist if the patient can still obey spoken commands. In this lightly sedated state, whilst in the left lateral position, the patient is asked to open his mouth. Should he have teeth, then a plastic mouthguard is inserted between them to protect the endoscope from damage by the teeth. The tip of the endoscope to be passed is then placed in the back of the mouth and gently pushed into the hypopharynx. At this stage, the patient is requested to make a swallowing action which carries the tip of the endoscope down into the upper

Table 3.1 Disorders in which endoscopy is superior to radiology in diagnosis and therapy

Reflux oesophagitis
Oesophageal varices
Upper gastrointestinal haemorrhage
Biopsy of suspect lesions
Radiologically negative dyspepsia
Therapeutic procedures

Table 3.2   Best tests in oesophageal, stomach and duodenal disease

Oesophagus	Barium meal
	and
	Endoscopy with biopsies
	Sometimes: pH studies
	motility studies
Stomach	Barium meal
	and
	Endoscopy with biopsies
	Sometimes measure: gastric acid output
	serum intrinsic factor
	vitamin B_{12}
	parietal cell antibodies
	gastrin
Duodenum	Barium meal
	or
	Endoscopy

oesophagus. The external light source and suction are then switched on to provide these services to the endoscope.

Using an end-viewing or oblique-viewing instrument, the endoscopist will be able to inspect the lumen of the oesophagus from the level of the throat all the way to the mucosal change where the stomach starts. The oesophagus is a long regular tube and this configuration can be readily identified from within. Normally, the endoscopist can also detect the regular peristaltic contractions, in addition to visualizing cardiac pulsation which is transmitted through the wall of the oesophagus. The oesophageal mucosa is a delicate pink colour and any retained oesophageal secretions are normally clear in colour and contain no blood. During the inspection, changes in the oesophagus, for example colour of the mucosa, the presence of abnormal mucosa as found in tumours or oesophagitis may be visualized. In the lower oesophagus, strictures may be present and the saccular out-pouching of a hiatus hernia may be seen. Rarely, the submucosal distortion of oesophageal varices may be noticed. If there has been excessive vomiting then a small tear in the mucosal lining may be present at the cardio–oesophageal junction. This is called a Mallory–Weiss tear.

The cardio–oesophageal junction is situated 38–45 cm from the incisor teeth. The narrow tube of the oesophagus passes at this level into the much larger cavity of the body of the stomach. At first, orientation may be difficult in this area. It is necessary to inflate the stomach with air and to aspirate any residual gastric contents before good mucosal views can be obtained. Once this has been done, it is usually possible to see prominent mucosal folds on one wall of the stomach. These are the folds of the greater curvature of the stomach and the endoscopist uses these for orientation (Fig. 3.7). Following them downwards leads to the antrum of the body of the stomach and the exist from the stomach to the duodenum, called the pylorus. Opposite the greater curve is the

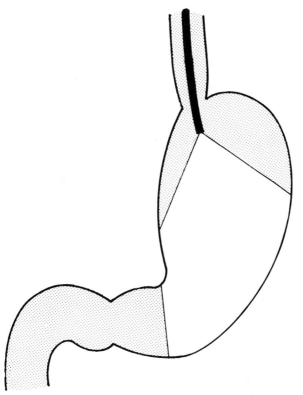

Fig. 3.7 *Typical view of body of stomach with an end-viewing instrument.*

lesser curve of the stomach which is featureless and carries no large folds. It ends at the incisura or angulus where the antrum starts. During inspection of the gastric cavity, the endoscopist will be inspecting the mucosa (of the stomach) for the presence of ulcers, irregularities, bleeding sites and malignant change. Once the tip of the endoscope is in the antrum, the nature of the peristaltic waves passing towards the pylorus should be inspected and the shape and contractability of the pylorus observed. Shallow ulcers on the rim of the pylorus are quite common (Fig. 3.8).

In this routine inspection of the stomach it is sometimes difficult to visualize the high lesser curve and the fundus of the body of the stomach. Modern end-viewing gastroscopes have greatly reduced this problem since they have such flexibility of the distal tip that they can be turned upwards sufficiently far to inspect these blind areas from below. In the antrum, this applies also to the antral aspect of the incisura on the lesser curve of the stomach (Fig. 3.9).

Once the inspection of the stomach has been completed, the endoscopist can pass through the pylorus into the first part of the duodenum. This is the commonest site of duodenal ulcers which may occur at any site within it. Ulcers may vary in size from tiny shallow erosions barely visible even with the endoscope,

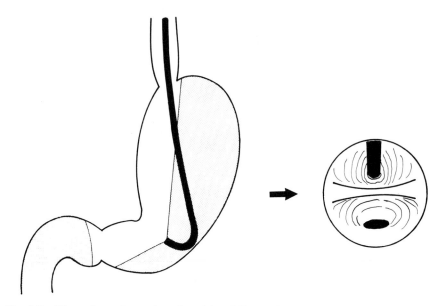

Fig. 3.8   *View of angulus and cardia with a 'U' turn deep in the antrum.*

to large necrotic areas which may be bleeding vigorously from an artery in the base of the ulcer. In this area, the endoscopist is required to make a thorough inspection of all aspects of the mucosa before negotiating into the more distal part of the duodenum round a prominent mucosal structure called the superior duodenal fold. Once past this fold, the endoscopist is once again looking into a tubular structure, the second part of the duodenum. It is differentiated from the body of the stomach by concentric mucosal folds, the valulae conniventes. Because bile is usually present in the duodenum, the mucosa has a yellowish or brownish colour which is not apparent in the stomach. On the medial wall of this part of the duodenum, it is usually possible to see the pimple-like structure, the ampulla of Vater, where the pancreatic and common bile ducts exit into the duodenum. A prominent ridge, the longitudinal fold, can also be identified leading towards the ampulla.

The abnormalities which the endoscopist will be looking for in this area are distortion of the tube-like structure of the duodenum due to external compression, the presence of ulcers in the immediate post-bulbar area and abnormalities of the ampulla of Vater. Once inspection has excluded these abnormalities the endoscopist may proceed down the second part of the duodenum to the next bend, where the third part of the duodenum may be entered. With conventional instruments this is the limit of upper gastrointestinal inspection.

Endoscopic biopsy

If abnormal mucosal features have been detected at any level in the upper gastrointestinal tract, then mucosal biopsies of the area in question may be

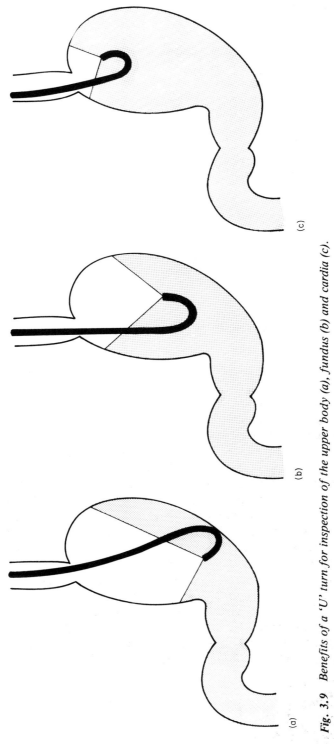

Fig. 3.9 *Benefits of a 'U' turn for inspection of the upper body (a), fundus (b) and cardia (c).*

obtained by biopsy forceps which can be passed down the channel of the endoscope. A whole range of biopsy forceps exist with different shaped jaws and
sometimes containing a central spike. The endoscopist advances the biopsy
forceps down the biopsy channel of the instrument until he can see that they will
impinge on the area of mucosa that he wishes to biopsy. The endoscopy assistant often controls the handle which opens and closes the forceps externally.
Multiple biopsies of suspicious areas should be obtained thus improving the
accuracy of histopathological interpretation (Fig. 3.10).

Brush cytology

Some endoscopic units are fortunate enough to have cytological techniques
available to them. Cytology provides an extra degree of accuracy in pathological assessment. It is best to obtain cytology specimens using a sheath brush
which can be passed down the channel of the endoscope in exactly the same way
as biopsy forceps. Once in line with the suspicious mucosal area, the brush can
be protruded beyond its sheath and rubbed across the mucosa. After retraction
of the brush into the sheath, the complete assembly is withdrawn from the
endoscope and thin smears of cells are made on clean microsope slides. To
preserve the cellular structures, the smears should then be sprayed with a
cellular fixative. Special slide carriers are made to prevent damage to
microscope slides in transit to the Cytopathology laboratory. Once in the

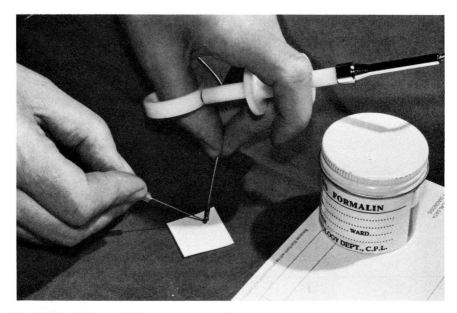

Fig. 3.10 *Endoscopic biopsy: removal of specimen from forceps to card prior to*
immersion in formalin.

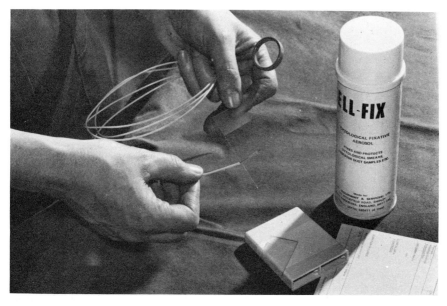

Fig. 3.11 *Endoscopic brush cytology: making slides prior to fixing with aerosol slide fixative.*

laboratory, cytology slides from the gastrointestinal tract are dealt with in much the same way as the smears for cervical cytology from the Gynaecology department (Fig. 3.11).

Large biopsies

If the endoscopist finds a large tumour mass or a polyp in the upper gastro-intestinal tract during his inspection, it is possible to obtain a large biopsy or even the complete polyp by diathermic excision using a snare loop and an external monopolar diathermy source.

Therapeutic Endoscopy

Oesophageal dilatation (Fig. 3.12)

Benign strictures of the oesophagus can be dilated using endoscopic techniques. The commonest of these is to use the Eder-Puestow system of metal olives which may be screwed onto a flexible wand. The olives are of progressively increasing size and are rail-roaded over a fine guide-wire which has previously been placed endoscopically through the strictured area. Radiological control is not always necessary but may be beneficial in some cases if the stricture is extremely tight. During the procedure, the endoscopy assistant has an important

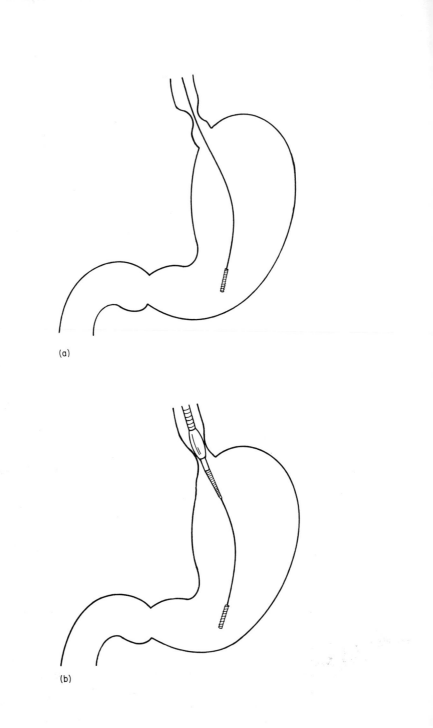

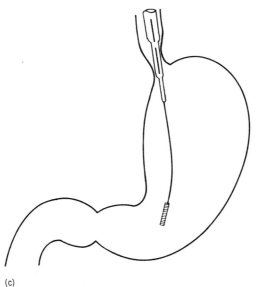

(c)

Fig. 3.12 *(a) Guide-wire placed in body of stomach. (b) Dilatation with Eder-Puestow dilator. (c) Dilatation with Celestin stepped dilator.*

part to play, ensuring that the patient's lips and tongue are not being damaged and that the guide-wire remains in a stable position. An assistant is also required to assemble the dilatation equipment and assist during the procedure.

An alternative to this technique is the use of Celestin's stepped dilator which is also passed over a guide-wire previously placed endoscopically through the oesophageal stricture. The advantage of this stepped dilator is that only two 'passes' through the pharynx are necessary and the stricture is dilated by progressive passage of increasing-sized steps through the stricture. A slight disadvantage of this alternative procedure is that by the time the biggest step of the dilator is through the stricture, the tip of the dilator is well down into the body of the stomach.

Oesophageal intubation (Fig. 3.13)

Where the lumen of the oesophagus is partially occluded by malignant tumour, the endoscopist can help the patient in a number of ways. In the first instance, it is usually possible to place a feeding tube through the narrowed area under endoscopic vision to maintain nutrition. If the case is considered inoperable, then prosthetic palliation may be undertaken with an endoscopic technique. In these procedures the malignant stricture is initially dilated as described above for benign stricture dilatation. Afterwards, a tube prosthesis may be inserted into the strictured area using a carrier device which grips the prosthetic tube tightly so that it may be inserted into the stricture under radiological control. The carrier device must have the ability to disengage from the prosthetic tube so that the tube remains in place across the stricture when the carrier is withdrawn.

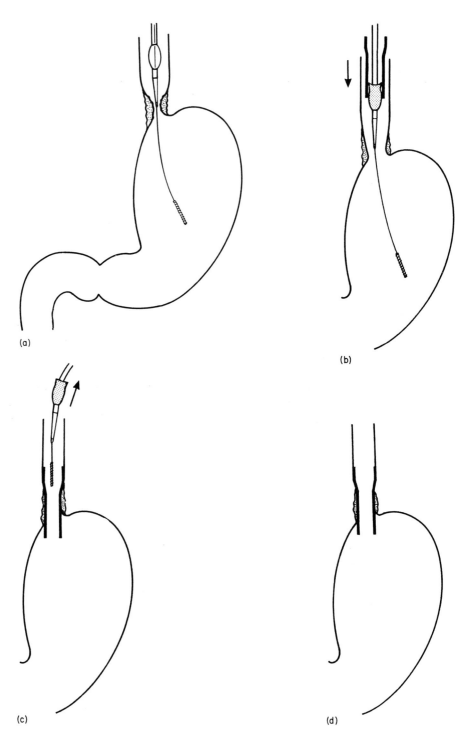

Fig. 3.13 *The stages of palliative oesophageal prosthesis insertion. (a) Dilatation, (b) insertion of prosthesis, (c) withdrawal of insertion system, and (d) prosthesis in situ.*

The systems which are currently available for this procedure include the KeyMed 'Nottingham' introducer for use with Atkinson prosthetic tubes or the Medoc Bristol system for insertion of Celestin Pulsion tubes.

Oesophageal sclerotherapy (Fig. 3.14)

In the past ten years, techniques have been developed and improved to produce a simple method of sclerotherapy of oesophageal varices using fibreoptic endoscopes. The basic principle of the technique requires the use of an end-viewing or oblique-viewing endoscope through which the oesophageal varices may be visualized and down the biopsy channel of which may be passed a flexible needle carrier with retractable needle. Oesophageal varices may then be injected with a sclerosant such as ethanolamine oleate or 3% sodium tetradecyl sulphate. The technique of individual endoscopists varies considerably. Some have a preference for general anaesthesia whilst others are happy to undertake sclerotherapy under light sedation. An overtube with a lateral orifice may be slid over the endoscope so that the varices protrude into the lumen through the orifice rendering them more readily visible. The endoscopy assistant has an important role in checking that the sclerotherapy needle is in good working order and fits the chosen endoscope. Under the supervision of the endoscopist, syringes will be primed with sclerosant. Protective spectacles may be worn to avoid splashing of the sclerosant into the eye as it can cause irritation. The assistant may inject the sclerosant on instruction from the endoscopist. Once the varices have been injected, the patient must be kept under observation for several hours to identify signs of post-procedural haemorrhage. Repeat endoscopic inspection and

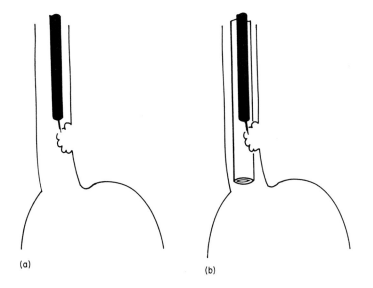

(a)

(b)

Fig. 3.14 *Endoscopic sclerotherapy technique. (a) Without overtube and (b) with overtube.*

sclerotherapy of residual varices is usually performed during the next few weeks until all varices are seen to be eradicated. Check endoscopy is thereafter undertaken every three months.

Endoscopy and radiation

The 10-day rule

A large number of investigations in gastroenterology involve exposing the patient to radiation by radiological screening or by administering a radioactive isotope and on some occasions both.

It is important to observe the Code of Practice for the Protection of Persons against Ionizing Radiations arising from Medical and Dental Use (DHSS, published by HMSO)* with particular reference to sections 7–7.3.1. and 7.3.2.:

'7.3.1.: In all women of reproductive capacity, the clinician requesting the examination should consider the possibility of an early stage of pregnancy. The date of the last menstrual period should be entered on the request form and it is the responsibility of the clinician requesting the examination to ascertain this. To reduce the likelihood of irradiation of a pregnancy, examinations should, if practicable, be carried out within 10 days following the first day of the menstrual period.

7.3.2.: Special precautions should be adopted in the radiography of women known to be pregnant. Only absolutely essential examinations should be carried out during pregnancy and particular care should be taken to minimise irradiation of the foetus.'

This is referred to throughout the book as 'The 10-Day Rule'.

Radiation hazard practice

Radiation can harm patients, staff and endoscopes. Patients must be given the correct protection such as lead sheeting over the gonads or ovaries and uterus. Only the minimum amount of screening should be used. Staff must wear protective clothing and regular monitoring of the radiation exposure of staff is required. Endoscopes should not be exposed longer than required as radiation can cause yellowing of the fibre bundles.

* Reproduced with the permission of the Controller of Her Majesty's Stationery Office.

Drug list

UK		USA	
Generic	Trade	Generic	Trade
Atropine	—	Atropine	—
Diazepam	Valium	Diazepam	Valium
	Diazemuls		
Fentanyl	Sublimaze	Fentanyl	Sublimaze
Pentazocine	Fortral	Pentazocine	Talwin
Pethidine	—	Meperidine	Demerol
Chlormethiazole	Heminevrin	Chlormethiazole	—
Naloxone	Narcan	Naloxone	Narcan
Metoclopramide	Maxolon	Metoclopramide	Reglan Injectable
	Primperan		Maxeran
Hyoscine butyl-bromide	Buscopan	Butylscopolamine	—
Sodium tetradecyl sulphate	STD	Sodium tetradecyl sulphate	Sotradecol
Ethanolamine oleate	—	Ethanolamine oleate	—
Hydrochloric acid	—	Hydrochloric acid	—
Sodium bicarbonate	—	Sodium bicarbonate	—
Glucagon	—	Glucagon	—
Secretin	—	Secretin	—
Pancreozymin	—	Pancreozymin	—
Mannitol	Osmitrol	Mannitol	Osmitrol
Pilocarpine	—	Pilocarpine	—
Magnesium sulphate	—	Magnesium sulphate	—
Casein	—	Casein	—
Maize Oil	—	Corn Oil	—
Dextrose	—	Dextrose	—
Pentagastrin	Peptavlon	Pentagastrin	Peptavlon
Vasopressin	Pitressin	Vasopressin	Pitressin

NURSING CARE DURING INVESTIGATION AND THERAPEUTIC PROCEDURES

Care of the patient in routine oesophagogastroduodenoscopy (OGD)

Check list

Endoscope of choice − an end-viewing gastroscope will be most commonly used but a side-viewing instrument should be available

Endoscopy trolley

continued

Accessories: biopsy forceps
               cytology brush
               cleaning brush
               camera
Light source
Water bottle and connecting tube
Sterile distilled water
Suction apparatus (2 units)
Aspiration catheters
Polythene tubing
Mouth guard
Drugs: premedication
      local anaesthesia
      sedation
      anticholinergic drugs
Needles
Syringes
Alcohol wipes
Intravenous cannulae
Adhesive tape
Gauze swabs
Lubricant
Disposable gloves
Histology specimen containers – ground glass or squares of card
Cytology fixative and slides with carriers
Histology request forms
Endoscopy report form

Consent

Advised written consent is required. This is best obtained by the doctor who is referring the patient for the procedure. Specially designed forms may be used or routine operation consent forms, depending on hospital practice and the clinician's preference.

Letter of appointment

This can be given or sent to outpatients and ought to contain the following relevant information:

A brief explanation of the procedure and instructions about fasting prior to arrival.
Date of appointment
Time of appointment
Location of department
A warning about the effects of any sedation to be used

A reference to the need for transport and a relative to accompany patient home

A telephone number, so that the patient may clarify any queries or alter the appointment if it is not convenient.

On arrival of the patient

The nurse should check that the letter has been understood and its contents adhered to

The consent form is checked

An identity bracelet is provided for the patient stating the name and hospital number

The patient's personal property is put in a safe place

Before any endoscopy examination, dentures must be removed, stored in a container and labelled with the patient's name and hospital number

Outdoor clothing is removed and a hospital gown provided in order to make the patient comfortable and protect the patient's own clothing from secretions or vomitus

Preparation of the patient

Instructions will have already been given to ensure that the patient has fasted for a minimum of four hours prior to endoscopy, as it is important the stomach is empty prior to the procedure. If there is a history of vomiting or the patient is known to have a degree of pyloric hold-up, it may be necessary to pass a nasogastric tube to aspirate stomach contents. A conventional stomach wash-out is seldom necessary as patients with copious stomach contents are unsuitable for endoscopy due to the risk of vomiting and inhalation of stomach contents.

For special circumstances see Chapter 8.

A careful check on the patient's mouth is required. Dentures are removed and any caps, loose teeth and dental caries are noted. If there is evidence of loose teeth, the endoscopist should be warned as these can be dislodged during the procedure and may be swallowed or inhaled. Sharp irregular teeth can also damage the endoscope and the endoscopist's fingers. A MOUTH GUARD MUST BE PROVIDED.

A history of drugs and allergies should be obtained and the hospital policy for these strictly adhered to.

When the patient is settled in bed or on a trolley, the premedication may be given. Atropine 0.6 mg i.m. is the most likely premedication but a premedication is not essential. Atropine helps to dry mouth secretions and also reduces gastric secretions, which facilitates the endoscopist's examination.

The notes and radiographs must be available and should accompany the patient into the endoscopy room.

During the procedure

The nurse and endoscopist on receiving the patient for examination will repeat the information about the procedure and reassure the patient.

Local anaesthetic may be used to numb the patient's throat. This can either be by lozenges (which should have been given to the patient at the time of pre-medication), gargle or spray. These should be given only if the patient is known to have no allergic reaction to them.

The patient is put comfortably into the left lateral position, with one pillow under the head ensuring the shoulder is not on the pillow, knees bent upwards and a pillow placed behind the patient's back to give support. The nurse should ensure that this position is maintained throughout the procedure as an alteration to the position can affect the endoscopist's view and may put the patient at risk if coughing or vomiting occurs.

Sedation of choice is administered by the endoscopist. The sedation is given *slowly* and titrated according to age, physical condition and observed patient response. Intravenous naloxone (Narcan) should be available to reverse the effect of sedation by pethidine.

The mouth guard may be either slipped onto the endoscope ready to be inserted by the endoscopist after the endoscope is in a satisfactory position, or it may be placed between the patient's teeth or gums while the sedation is being administered and the patient can be asked to keep it in position.

Intubation

The endoscope is lubricated with either a water-soluble lubricant or with a wet swab. The endoscope is passed by the endoscopist using the method of choice. The light source and suction pump are switched on and patient suction readily available to remove excess secretions or vomitus from the mouth as necessary.

The nurse reassures the patient, keeps a check of vital functions and ensures the correct position is maintained. She must remember the endoscopist is engrossed with the technical aspects of the procedure and the nurse is responsible for monitoring the patient's condition.

Pathology

The nurse will be required to provide the biopsy forceps and assist in the collection of histology and cytology specimens. Careful records of specimens obtained and the completion of the appropriate forms are important to prevent errors occurring.

Photography

When required, a camera must be provided with film and the number of photographs recorded with patient details to ensure satisfactory use of the photographs.

Documentation

After the procedure the nurse is required to ensure that a report is completed and inserted into the patient's notes. Depending on the system used, copies may be stored in the department and/or sent to the patient's general practitioner.

Information about patients and procedures may also be recorded in the department books or ledgers in order to provide records for statistics and research purposes. Follow-up plans may also be made at this stage. For patient information and documentation see Appendix B.

Recovery

The patient is moved to a recovery area and observed while recovering from the procedure (Fig. 3.15).

After the procedure

During endoscopy gastric insufflation is essential to improve the field of view. If the air is not aspirated by the endoscopist at the end of the procedure, this may give rise to discomfort or pain.

An adequate period should elapse before eating and drinking recommences in order to allow the effect of local anaesthesia to wear off.

The long term effects of sedation will have already been explained to the patient. If i.v. diazepam is used, the effects can last as long as 36 hours. Warnings about possible self-injury and the dangers of alcohol, driving and working with machinery must be repeated before the patient is discharged.

Complications of endoscopy

The possible effects of some drugs can be dangerous with regard to respiratory and cardiovascular problems and the properties of the drugs in use in the department should be fully understood by the nurse.

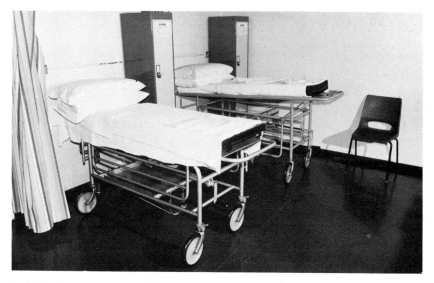

Fig. 3.15   Recovery area with lockers for patients' property and showing (right) head-down facility on patient trolley.

Any abdominal pain will be mostly due to the air insufflation and therefore transient.

Local thrombophlebitis is a known complication of some types of intravenous drugs and the endoscopist should be aware of methods to minimize this problem by correction injection using barbotage or using less irritant types of the drug.

Haemorrhage may occur after biopsy or the procedure may promote rebleeding in an acute situation such as an active ulcer or oesophageal varices.

Aspiration pneumonia may occur due to inhalation of gastric contents.

Perforation may occur due to incorrect intubation technique or by using biopsy forceps in a situation such as a deep penetrating gastric ulcer.

Care of the patient during oesophageal dilatation

At least two nurses are required to assist to ensure this procedure is carried out safely and satisfactorily.

Check list

A slim end-viewing or oblique-viewing gastroscope will be required

Trolley, suction, accessories as for routine OGD

Biopsy/brushings for histology/cytology may be required if the pathology has not already been confirmed at earlier endoscopy or if repeat investigations are required

Dilatation equipment of choice

Protective glasses for staff − the end of the guide-wire is sharp and can cause eye injuries

Arrange radiology facilities if required

Check 10-day rule

Preparation

On receiving the patient, the nurse will explain the procedure and ensure it has been understood. She must check that informed written consent has been obtained by the referring clinician.

The patient is prepared as for routine OGD. Depending on the patient's condition and the preference of the clinician, admission for one or two nights may be required.

The patient is fasted for a minimum of four hours. Intravenous parenteral nutrition may have been required pre-operatively and on arrival for the procedure, this must be checked to ensure that it is functioning satisfactorily.

Explanation should be given regarding the after-effects of the procedure and the patient reassured as to the benefits of the dilatation.

The procedure may take place in the Radiology department or Gastroenterology department. Dentures are removed and local anaesthetic is administered. Discomfort during this procedure may be experienced in the throat and adequate local anaesthesia is essential.

The patient is positioned in the left lateral position with one pillow under the head and one at the patient's back. Should the dilators or tube introducers deviate from the mid-line during the procedure, perforation of the pharynx, oesophagus or stomach may occur. It is the duty of the nurse to ensure that the correct position is maintained throughout the procedure as the endoscopist will be concentrating on the technique.

Sedation is administered by the endoscopist. General anaesthesia is optional. Intravenous naloxone (Narcan) should be available. Resuscitation facilities should be at hand.

The patient's case notes and radiology must be available and it is helpful to have the recent barium swallow films on the viewing box where they can be seen during the procedure.

The procedure for oesophageal dilatation

Using Eder—Puestow dilators

The endoscopist passes the end-viewing gastroscope as for normal OGD examination. If a slim gastroscope is used it may be possible to pass this through the stricture but it could still be desirable to proceed with dilatation. The bigger diameter gastroscope may be too large to pass through the stricture and it will then be necessary to proceed to dilatation. In simple peptic strictures the gastroscope may in itself act as a dilator and it will not be necessary to proceed to dilatation.

One assistant now controls the patient's head and reassures the patient. The second assistant assembles the dilators and holds the guide-wire taught when requested by the endoscopist.

After assessing the degree of stricture, the endoscopist passes the guide-wire through the biopsy channel of the gastroscope and either

(1) manipulates the end of the wire into a safe place in the body of the stomach by direct endoscopic view, or

(2) manipulates it into place under radiological control.

The proximal end of the wire is aligned to a fixed point (in the room) and this is referred to throughout the procedure.

The gastroscope is withdrawn, whilst the endoscopist maintains the wire correctly positioned in the stomach. The wire is held firmly at the mouth by the assistant at the patient's head.

The gastroscope is quickly checked for correct functioning, rinsed, wiped dry and left on the trolley for further use.

The endoscopist holds the wire and requests the assembled dilator with the olive of choice mounted.

The endoscopist passes the dilator over the guide wire which is held firmly in position by the assistant, and the olive dilates up the stricture. The olives are changed in increasing size until the desired degree of dilatation is obtained.

The wire is removed with the last olive. The endoscopist may pass the gastroscope to check the condition of the mucosa and examine the remainder of the oesophagus, stomach and duodenum if desired.

Diligent use of mouth aspiration is necessary throughout this procedure since it may give rise to accumulation of secretions or regurgitated gastric contents in the patient's mouth.

Routine post-endoscopy care is given after dilatation. A chest radiograph may be performed but is not essential. The patient may experience transient retrosternal discomfort or soreness of the throat.

Stepped dilatation system

Check list

As for routine gastrointestinal endoscopy plus:
Celestin stepped dilators
Guide-wire
Water tray with iced water
If radiological screening is used, the 10-day rule must be checked and observed as appropriate

---

Procedure

This is similar to Eder–Puestow dilatation. The guide-wire is passed through the suction/biopsy channel of the endoscope and the endoscope is withdrawn. One nurse looks after the patient and holds the guide-wire at the mouth. The second nurse passes the chilled dilators to the endoscopist and holds the guide-wire taught during dilatation. The dilators are passed gently over the guide-wire and gradual dilatation of the oesophageal stricture obtained. The guide-wire is withdrawn with the last dilator and the patient made comfortable. Postprocedural care is the same as that for Eder–Puestow dilatation.

Complications of oesophageal dilatation

These are as for routine OGD plus possible perforation of pharynx, oesophagus and stomach. Perforation may occur if the guide-wire is misplaced or damaged, causing injury to the mucosa. Observation for development of surgical emphysema, with or without chest radiology, is important. Perforation may be treated conservatively with intravenous infusion, gastric aspiration, bed rest and routine observations.

Oesophageal intubation

Nursing care

At least two nurses are required to assist to ensure this procedure is carried out safely and satisfactorily.

Check list

As for oesophageal dilatation plus:
   Prosthesis of choice: Celestin Pulsion Endo-Oesophageal Prosthesis
                         Atkinson's Oesophageal Prosthesis
   Appropriate introducing system
   It may be necessary to cut the prosthesis to fit the lesion so sharp scissors will
also be required
   A tape measure should be available

Procedure for oesophageal intubation

Radiological control is essential for this procedure. Intubation can only take place
after complete dilatation of the malignant stricture. Although the procedure may
be conducted under light sedation, some endoscopists prefer general anaesthesia.
In the UK, the Nottingham Intubation system is commonly used in conjunction
with the Eder–Puestow dilators, whilst the Celestin dilatation and intubation
systems are a suitable alternative. In the USA, the Worth-Boyce system is most
frequently used. Dilatation should normally be conducted to 48F gauge to aid
tube placement, but in some cases even greater dilatation may be required.

After dilatation the endoscopist will establish the length of the lesion to be
straddled and select a suitable prosthesis which may be cut to the correct size if
necessary. The prosthesis should be mounted on the Nottingham Introducer
which consists of inner and outer shafts, a Delrin expanding olive and a flexible
leading tip. The technique depends upon expansion of the Delrin olive within
the prosthesis where it is held in position by the bayonet locking system.

The introducer and prosthesis are passed over the guide-wire which has been
left in position after dilatation, and the position of the prosthesis in the oesophagus is confirmed by radiology. The Delrin olive-expanding system is released
and with the aid of radiology it is possible to ensure that the prosthesis remains in
the correct position straddling the lesion. It may be necessary at this point to use
the rammer. The rammer may be rendered malleable by placing it in hot water. It
should be placed over the introducing system while it is *in situ* and pushed down
until it comes in contact with the proximal funnel of the prosthesis. The
introducer may be withdrawn while the rammer is held in position and it can be
observed radiologically that the radio-opaque marker on the prosthesis remains
static. Alternatively, the rammer can be used after the introducer is withdrawn to
push the prosthesis firmly home under radiological control (Fig. 3.16).

Celestin Pulsion Intubation System

Mandril set

Bristol Balloon Introducer (SB) is used for intubation of the Celestin Pulsion
tube.

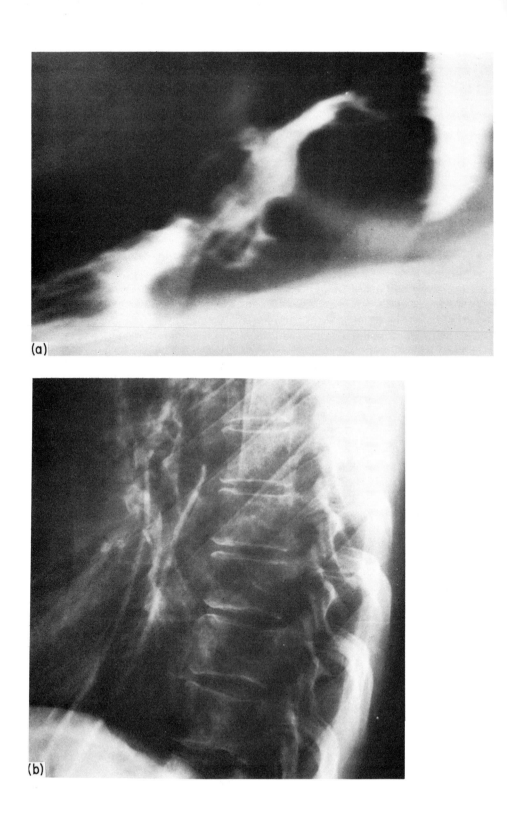

It is important that the balloon should be dry at all times and be protected from contamination with lubricants as otherwise it will slip and intubation will fail.

The Bristol Balloon Introducer (SB) is dependent on the use of a mandril that carries the introducer and stiffens it.

The mandril is in 2 parts: a shaft with a female thread at one end and a bullet-shaped head mounted on a short stem carrying a male thread for screwing into the shaft.

The shaft of the mandril is inserted into the lumen at the long end of the introducer and pushed until it abuts firmly a shoulder at the lower, or shorter end of the introducer.

The stem of the bullet-head is now pushed through the lumen of the shorter end and screwed fully into the shaft of the mandril. Ensure that this manoeuvre has been achieved by trying to distract the shaft from the bullet-head.

Empty the balloon of all air and slip the introducer into the pulsion tube until the bullet-head just projects beyond its lower end.

Using a 20 ml syringe, inflate with 10–15 ml of air until the balloon securely grips the inside walls of the tube and cannot be pulled out.

Remove the syringe from the check valve.

Thoroughly lubricate the bullet-head and the lower end of the pulsion tube to include the skirt and the area above it and slide the fully mounted set over the guide-wire already threaded through the stricture which has been carefully dilated to 48F and its distance from the incisor teeth noted.

The intubation set is already in the operator's right hand while the left index finger retracts the patient's tongue forward and guides the introducer past the pharynx into the oesophagus. Gentle pressure is exerted until the funnel of the tube is below the pharynx when the index finger can be withdrawn.

Continue to apply pressure until the tube is felt to engage the stricture, the skirt will also be felt to engage the stricture, and pressure is continued until the funnel reaches the lesion, when the tube can no longer be advanced and at which time the graduation figure on the introducer should correspond to the distance of the stricture from the incisor teeth.

Pressure is relaxed, at which time the introducer will move up a few centimetres. Deflate the balloon and by a side-to-side rotating movement, recall the introducer until it is fully removed.

If a small-bore fibrescope is available it may be passed through the prosthesis and the oesophagus and stomach examined.

Fibrescopic set

Bristol Balloon Introducer (FB) is used for intubation of the Celestin Pulsion tube.

Fig. 3.16 *Palliative prosthetic insertion in carcinoma of oesophagus. (a) Pre-intubation and (b) post-intubation.*

Method of use

It is important that the balloon should be dry at all times, and be protected from contamination with lubricants as otherwise it will slip and inbubation will fail.

The Bristol Balloon Introducer (FB) for direct visual insertion of the Celestin Pulsion tube is dependent upon the use of an end-viewing fibrescope with a diameter of 10.5 mm or less.

Procedure

Having already biopsied and dilated the stricture to 48F gauge, the introducer and pulsion tube are slipped over the endoscope in that order. The funnel of the tube is made to engage the balloon which is then inflated to its maximum to grip the funnel firmly.

The endoscope beyond the tube is generously lubricated and endoscopy repeated until the tip of the instrument lies just above the dilated stricture. The introducer and tube are now pushed down until the latter is made to engage the stricture. Under direct vision and using steady pressure, the tube is navigated through the stricture until the funnel arrests further movement. At this point, the balloon end of the introducer will come into view. The balloon is now deflated and the introducer removed.

To remove a prosthesis using either system, the introducer is pushed into the prosthesis and the system expanded appropriately. By a steady pull, the prosthesis can be removed.

Post-procedural patient care

The patient is given routine post-endoscopy care but should be admitted for at least one night after the procedure. The patient is nursed with 2–3 pillows to prevent reflux of gastric contents and should be advised to continue this practice at home. Fluids may be given 4–6 hours after intubation. Oesophageal perforation should be excluded and the position of the tube checked the following day by chest radiology.

A semi-solid diet can be started in 24 hours. It is important that solids are chewed at least twice as long as is done normally. Carbonated drinks sipped during and after meals are important as they keep the tube clear. Written instructions should be given to the patient to take home.

The gastroenterology nurse must reassure the patient about the benefits of the tube and offer the necessary support for a terminally ill patient. It is helpful to provide a telephone number to which the patient can resort in the event of blockage or dislodgement of the tube.

The help of the dietitian can be enlisted to give advice on foods which can be readily swallowed and how to use a liquidizer or pulveriser to the best and most interesting dietary advantage.

Complications for oesophageal intubation

These are as for routine OGD with the possibility of perforation during the dilatation procedure and the added risk of splitting of the oesophageal wall during intubation. Observation and nursing care as for oesophageal dilatation are essential. Gastro-oesophageal reflux may be a problem, but can be minimized by elevation of the bed-head and treatment with anti-reflux therapy.

Pneumatic dilatation of the oesophagus

Nursing care

At least two nurses are required to assist to ensure this procedure is carried out safely and satisfactorily.

Check list

As for oesophagoscopy plus:
  Dilatation equipment of choice: e.g. Rider–Moeller
  Brown–McHardy

Procedure

The patient is oesophagoscoped and the guide-wire positioned under endoscopic and fluoroscopic control, depending on the ease with which the endoscopist can visualize the aperture at the strictured area.

The endoscope is removed, ensuring the guide-wire remains in the correct position. The dilator is passed over the guide-wire and visualized by fluoroscopy. The bag is inflated with air by a standard rubber bulb and the pressure measured by manometry. A pressure of $9-12$ lb inch^{-2} for $4-6$ seconds should be effective but fluoroscopic appearances and pain must also be considered.

Post-procedural patient care

The patient is given post-endoscopy care but should be admitted for at least one night after the procedure. Pain should subside but if it persists, medical staff should be informed. It is preferable for the patient to be nursed with $2-3$ pillows to prevent reflux of gastric contents. A chest radiograph should be taken the following day and a check barium swallow may be given after 48 hours to ascertain the success of the procedure. It may be necessary to perform repeat dilatations in order to produce a satisfactory effect.

Complications

Complications which are possible though rare are perforation and haemorrhage. Others which may occur owing to the increase in the oesophageal diameter are reflux of gastric contents and aspiration of gastric contents.

With correct positioning of the patient and good nursing care these complications may be avoided.

Sclerotherapy

At least two nurses are required for this procedure.

Check list

As for routine fibreoptic oesophagoscopy plus:
Sclerotherapy needle — depending on the endoscope to be used
Sclerosant of choice: sodium tetradecyl sulphate 3% w.v.
ethanolamine oleate
Syringes
Protective spectacles
An end-viewing or oblique-viewing endoscope may be used

Preparation of equipment

The needle should be disinfected or sterilized before use — as per method employed for other accessories in the department.

Small quantities of sclerosant can be drawn up ready for use. An injection size of 1–2 ml is usual and it may be easier to use small syringes to get accurate measurements and ensure easy injection of the sclerosant as the high viscosity of some substances can make this difficult.

Fill lumen of injection needle wearing gloves and spectacles, taking care to wrap gauze swabs round the connection between the syringe and needle to absorb any leak of sclerosant.

Procedure

This is as for routine fibreoptic oesophagoscopy with one nurse controlling the patient's head and paying particular attention to the patient's vital functions should there be active bleeding.

When the endoscopist has located the varices to be injected, the second nurse hands the loaded needle with syringe attached. The needle is passed through the endoscope in the same way as biopsy forceps.

The nurse will be required to advance and retract the needle and to inject the measured amount of sclerosant when asked by the endoscopist.

The patient may experience retrosternal discomfort and will require re-assurance that this is transient.

After the procedure, the patient should rest comfortably. Pulse and respiration rate should be checked and any changes reported to the physician.

The patient may be admitted for 24 hours post-procedure.

Complications of sclerotherapy

After the procedure the patient may complain of substernal pain which usually passes off spontaneously. Rarely, the pain may increase in severity and be accompanied by tachycardia, hypotension and fever. These features indicate the development of mediastinitis, secondary to extra-oesophageal injection or a small perforation. The doctor must be informed.

Occasionally the procedure will precipitate re-bleeding which may require the re-insertion of a Sengstaken–Blakemore tube, whilst ulceration of the oesophagus at the site of injection may eventually cause scarring and a stricture. Such strictures may be dilated with safety by conventional means.

Gastric polypectomy

Check list

As for routine OGD plus:
    Diathermy equipment − checked and working
    Snares to suit individual endoscope
    Retrieval instruments − graspers or basket for large polyps, or sputum trap in suction tubing for small polyps which may be aspirated via the suction channel of the endoscope

Procedure

This is as for routine OGD with the addition of the use of diathermy.

The patient diathermy plate is put in position. The diathermy system is connected up to the patient plate, snare and endoscope. The power is set to the endoscopist's requirement. The snare is passed through the suction/biopsy channel of the endoscope.

The polyp is excised by diathermic current and then may be removed from the stomach by whichever method is thought to be appropriate.

A check for bleeding is essential before the endoscopy is complete.

The patient's pulse and respiration rate are checked. An overnight stay may be necessary.

Complications of gastric polypectomy

This is as for routine OGD plus the possibility of bleeding from the site of excision. Routine observations should be carried out, and blood taken for group and save prior to the procedure.

The complications of diathermy may be avoided by ensuring the unit is functioning correctly (see Fig. 5.13) and all connections are secure. Care must be taken to avoid skin burns.

Foreign body removal

Check list

As for routine upper gastrointestinal endoscopy plus:
    Grasping and retrieval instruments

In some instances the conventional retrievers may be unsuitable and forceps, snares etc. may be used. In the case of sharp objects it is possible to use a wide bore rubber or polythene tube over the endoscope to protect the mucosa from the sharp edges of the object when it is being retrieved. The nurse is required to be inventive and calm during this procedure!

Procedure

The procedure should be conducted as for routine endoscopy.

The patient is required to be kept quiet and reassured. Extra sedation may be required and general anaesthesia may be necessary. Hyoscine butyl bromide (Buscopan) should be available to paralyse the gastrointestinal tract, thereby facilitating easier removal of the foreign body. It is important the situation is calm and there are no involuntary movements or sudden interruptions.

Post-procedure care

This will be as for routine endoscopy. If bleeding has resulted the clinical management will be as for the bleeding patient and may include surgical intervention.

Complications of foreign body removal

These are as for routine OGD plus perforation from sharp objects, but this may be minimized by use of an overtube (Fig. 3.17). Impaction of objects in the oesophagus is also possible, and foreign bodies may be dropped into the gastric lake by the retrieval instrument. If there is hypermobility of the upper gastro-intestinal tract, the foreign body may move rapidly down the gut during endoscopy and make retrieval impossible.

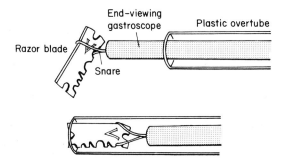

Fig. 3.17   Foreign body removal – extraction of sharp object using an overtube.

NON-ENDOSCOPIC DIAGNOSTIC PROCEDURES

Acid perfusion of the oesophagus

The differentiation of oesophageal from cardiac pain is often extremely difficult. A technique which helps in some way to do so is to perfuse the lower oesophagus with dilute hydrochloric acid. If, during this procedure, the patient develops pain identical to that experienced clinically, then it is further evidence that the oesophagus is the site of pain. The technique depends on the radiological placement of an oesophageal tube with its tip 8–10 cm above the cardio–oesophageal junction. A check lateral chest radiograph should be used to confirm the position. Thereafter, dilute hydrochloric acid may be dripped down the tube at a standard rate during the test phase. Sodium chloride (0.9%) or sodium bicarbonate infused at the same rate may be used as a control. Only pain produced with hydrochloric acid should be regarded as indicative of a positive test. The patient should not be aware of which solution is being infused at any one time and should be sitting in a relaxed atmosphere with attention diverted from the procedure itself. The major drawback of the procedure is the subjective interpretation of the patient's response.

Oesophageal pH and oesophageal manometry

These tests are in limited use in the UK. They are indicated in four main situations.

When the clinician needs to know whether a patient does or does not have significant gastro-oesophageal reflux

When the patient appears to have an oesophageal motility disorder but its nature, extent or cause is not clear

When it is necessary to determine whether obscure or atypical symptoms (e.g. chest pain) are or are not caused by an oesophageal disorder

When it is necessary to assess objectively the functional results of therapy, either medical or surgical

Oesophageal pH may be measured using a pH electrode or radiopill tethered at the face and located 8–10 cm above the cardia. Continuous monitoring of distal oesophageal pH can then be undertaken over a prolonged period. Under normal circumstances transient episodes of oesophageal reflux occur and the distal oesophageal pH quickly returns to normal. Under pathological circumstances, reflux episodes are more frequent and clearing less efficient. pH monitoring for prolonged periods, especially overnight, can reveal the pathological nature of these episodes.

Oesophageal manometry is the technique whereby oesophageal pressure may be recorded. It may be undertaken with an open-ended triple lumen tube system perfused with sodium chloride 0.9% or with closed balloons. In each case, the pressure changes are recorded via transducers onto a pen-recorder system. An additional test is to measure lower oesophageal sphincter pressure by a pull-through technique in which changes of pressure within the gastric fundus, lower and middle oesophagus are recorded. Reduced lower oesophageal sphincter pressure may contribute to a tendency to reflux. Again, the pressure recording system is via a transducer to a pen-recorder system.

Gastric acid analysis

The volume and concentration of acid secreted by the stomach may be measured by aspirating gastric contents and physical measurement. The performance of such a test enables the physician to assess the normality or abnormality of gastric acid secretion and has been used in the past to determine the best type of operation for recurrent peptic ulceration. Although its use for this purpose has largely been abandoned, the technique is still widely used to assess the adequacy of vagotomy in patients who have recurrent peptic ulceration post-operatively. Gastric acid secretion will either be stimulated by the injection of agents such as histamine or pentagastrin or alternatively the patient may be rendered mildly hypoglycaemic by injections of insulin (Hollander test). This latter technique stimulates gastric secretion via the vagus nerves and is used to assess their integrity. Combined injections have been used to provoke maximum gastric acid output. The procedures are performed on the previously starved patient in whom a nasogastric tube has been positioned in the body of the stomach. Thereafter, the left lateral position is maintained to facilitate collection of accumulated gastric secretion and an aspiration pump is used to collect the secretions in a time sequence both before (basal secretion) and after stimulation. The procedure is a tedious one for patients and its successful performance requires skilful attention to detail by the nurse or technician involved to ensure that all gastric secretion is collected and that the tube does not become blocked. If insulin is being used as the gastric stimulant then it is a wise precaution to monitor blood glucose levels throughout the procedure and to have intravenous dextrose available for use should the patient become profoundly hypoglycaemic.

Acid Perfusion of the Oesophagus

Check list

Solutions required from Pharmacy:
  1 litre hydrochloric acid 0.1 normal
  1 litre sodium bicarbonate 0.1 normal
  1 litre sodium chloride 0.9%
  I.V. infusion sets × 3, i.e. 1 per solution

Glass flasks with rubber stoppers are the preferred containers for these solutions

Other requirements:
  Nasogastric tube of choice or Foley Catheter size 18F
  Lubrication
  Gauze swabs
  Adhesive tape
  10 ml syringe – if using Foley Catheter
  Tissues
  Vomit towl
  A comfortable upright chair
  Magazines for the patient to read

Procedure

The patient will have fasted for 12 hours. On receiving the patient, the nurse will explain the procedure and ensure that it has been understood and check the 10-day rule where appropriate. Informed written consent must be obtained by the referring clinician and checked by the nurse. The patient's dentures should be removed in case of nausea and the patient seated comfortably on the chair. The tube to be used is lubricated and passed via the nose so that the tip is 8–10 cm above the diaphragm, after which the position should be checked radiologically.

Magazines are provided for distraction and the reactions of the patient to the procedure are observed closely. The infusion regime is as follows:

(1) Attach sodium chloride 0.9% to run through 15 drops per minute. 10 ml in 10 minutes

(2) Change to hydrochloric acid as above

(3) Change to sodium bicarbonate as above

(4) Attach sodium chloride 0.9% to run through at 30 drops per minute 20 ml in 10 minutes

(5) Change to hydrochloric acid as above

(6) Change to sodium bicarbonate as above

A positive test is obtained by pain produced by hydrochloric acid and relieved by sodium bicarbonate. False positives may occur with other fluids but do not indicate pain from reflux oesophagitis. A note should be recorded as to when pain occurs and the nature of the pain.

Alternatively, if a Foley Catheter is used, the balloon should be inflated after the infusion regime is completed. Should the patient experience tightening in the chest similar to the presenting symptoms, this too may indicate oesophageal disease.

At the end of the procedure remove the tube and make the patient comfortable. If not proceeding to endoscopy at the same visit, the patient may be allowed to eat and drink.

All disposable equipment used must be discarded.

Pentagastrin and Hollander tests

Check list

Nasogastric tube of choice – this must be radio-opaque, (e.g. Porges, Salem sump, Anderson AN10)

Lubricant (e.g. K-Y Jelly)

Gauze swabs

Adhesive tape

Receiver

Blue litmus paper

20 ml syringe for aspirating secretions

2 ml syringes and needles for injection of stimulants

continued

Pentagastrin (Peptavalon)
Soluble insulin
50% glucose solution
Optional: suction pump e.g. Cape Aspirating Table, Down's pump

Procedure for pentagastrin test

The patient fasts for 12 hours and is weighed on arrival. On receiving the patient, the nurse will explain the procedure, ensure that it has been understood and check the 10-day rule where appropriate. Informed written consent must be obtained by the referring clinician and checked by the nurse.

The patient's dentures are removed in case of nausea. When seated in an upright chair or in bed, the patient is asked to clear the nose and the tube is passed via the nose to a depth of 45–50 cm from the external nares and fixed comfortably with adhesive tape. The position of the tube should be checked radiologically and the tip visualized halfway down the greater curve of the stomach.

Aspirate is tested with litmus paper. Blue turning red indicates acid and therefore stomach contents. Overnight secretions are aspirated and discarded. The tube may be spiggotted or connected to continuous suction at a pressure of 3–5 cm Hg.

Basal secretion is collected over 30 minutes, measured and stored. Pentagastrin stimulation is now given. Dosage is 6 μg per kg body weight and it is given *intramuscularly*. Following this, gastric secretions are collected at 15 minutes intervals for four collections, i.e. over a period of one hour. If there is an indication that the tube may be blocked, air can be injected to clear it.

The five specimens are sent for analysis and the tube is removed. The patient is made comfortable and normal eating and drinking can commence if this is in accordance with the individual patient's care plan.

Procedure for Hollander test

This is as for the pentagastrin test until the basal collection period is completed, after which blood should be taken for fasting blood sugar estimation. Stimulation by insulin is now given. Dosage is 0.2 μg per kg body weight and the insulin is given *intravenously*.

Two full hours of gastric secretions are collected post-injection in 8 × 15 minute aliquots. The blood glucose level is checked at 30 minutes and 45 minutes post-injection. All samples are sent for analysis.

The tube is removed and the patient made comfortable. Normal eating and drinking may commence if this is in accordance with the individual patient's care plan.

Complications of Hollander test

Hypoglycaemia will occur after administration of insulin. This should be transient but if persistent or severe may require to be reversed with oral or intravenous glucose. The test must then be abandoned.

4

THE SMALL INTESTINE

ANATOMY

The small intestine is that portion of the digestive tract extending from the duodenojejunal junction to its termination at the ileocaecal valve which is the start of the large intestine. The total length of this tube-like structure is about six metres and it consists of two parts, the jejunum and the ileum. The jejunum is the more proximal part and passes imperceptibly into the ileum which forms the distal half of the small intestine. Both parts are mobile within the abdominal cavity, being attached to the posterior abdominal wall by a curtain of tissue called the mesentery. The ileum terminates distally in the ileocaecal valve where the small intestine enters the caecum, the first part of the large intestine or colon.

The major role of the small intestine is in the absorption of digestive products. A cross section reveals that it has four coats:

An outer or peritoneal layer
A muscular layer consisting of longitudinal and circular fibres
A submucosal or supportive layer
The mucosa

The mucosa is arranged in folds called valvulae conniventes. The effect of these folds is to greatly increase the surface area from which absorption can take place. The surface of the mucous membrane is covered with tiny hair-like projections called villi. These are specially adapted for the absorption of food into the bloodstream. The cells on their surface produce enzymes which are secreted into the intestinal juice and aid breakdown of digestive products. Each villus contains capillaries into which are absorbed the products of carbohydrate and protein digestion and a central lacteal vessel into which fats are absorbed (Fig. 4.1).

Aggregations of lymphoid tissue called Peyer's patches are found in the sub-mucosa of the ileum. These lymphoid aggregations seem to have a role in the

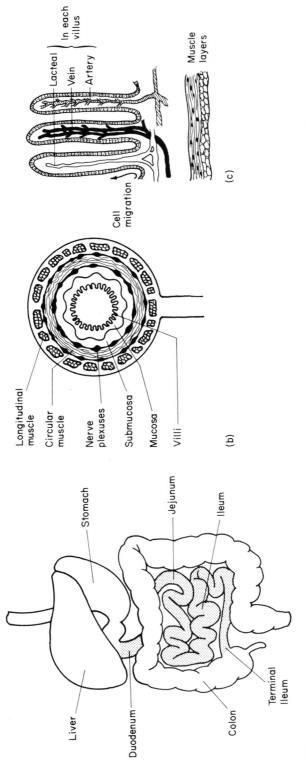

Fig. 4.1 (a) Components of the small intestine, note their relationship to other intra-abdominal organs. (b) Diagram of wall of small intestine. (c) Section through the wall.

prevention of absorption of bacteria and are especially important in typhoid fever when they become very inflamed.

The blood supply to the small intestine comes from the superior mesenteric artery which arises directly from the aorta. The superior mesenteric artery divides into a system of arcades of vessels which run in the mesentery and subdivide into a capillary network within the wall of the intestine. Venous blood from the small intestine drains into the superior mesenteric vein which carries blood containing absorbed products of digestion to the liver via the portal venous system.

PHYSIOLOGY

Within the lumen of the upper small intestine, food products continue to be broken down into smaller units of carbohydrate, protein and fat which are

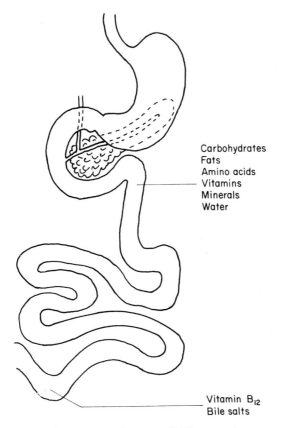

Carbohydrates
Fats
Amino acids
Vitamins
Minerals
Water

Vitamin B_{12}
Bile salts

Fig. 4.2 *Small intestinal absorptive function. Different substances are absorbed at different levels.*

capable of absorption at some stage during their passage through the small bowel. This process of digestion is further aided by the secretion of intestinal juice or succus entericus containing water, electrolytes and enzymes. The total volume of this intestinal juice secreted daily is about three litres, most of which is reabsorbed into the bloodstream either in the small bowel itself or more distally in the colon.

Absorption of digestive products into the bloodstream is aided by the mucosal folds and projections previously mentioned. Various levels of the small intestine are specially adapted to absorb different products of digestion (Fig. 4.2). Most electrolytes, vitamins, carbohydrates, proteins and fat products are absorbed in the proximal small bowel. The distal ileum is specially adapted to absorb vitamin B_{12} and to reabsorb bile salts. These differing levels for intestinal absorptive function take on added importance when diseases or surgical removal are considered, since it is possible that certain functions of the small intestine are affected whilst others remain intact.

Once the large particles of carbohydrate, protein and fat have been broken down into small units, they are actively absorbed through the surface of the villi of the small intestine either into the capillary loops within the villi or, in the case of fats, directly into the specialized lymphatic vessels called lacteals. Through these systems, products of digestion are conveyed to the liver or directly to the bloodstream for immediate utilization or storage.

PATHOLOGY (Fig. 4.3)

Malabsorption

The commonest end-result of disease of the small intestine is malabsorption of one or more essential nutrients, electrolytes, minerals or vitamins. The patient may present with diarrhoea, abdominal pain and distension, weight loss, anaemia or evidence of nutritional deficiency. Frequently, steatorrhoea is the presenting symptom. This is the passage of loose, pale, offensive-smelling stools which float on water. Sometimes the patient is anaemic due to a deficiency of iron, vitamin B_{12} or folic acid. Defective absorption of vitamin K may lead to haemorrhagic phenomena and multiple bruising. A low serum calcium may result in tetany, whilst prolonged defective absorption of vitamin D may lead to softening of the bones called osteomalacia (rickets in childhood). Other vitamin deficiencies may result in a sore tongue, cracking at the corners of the mouth or dry, rough scaly skin. Peripheral oedema may be the result of a low serum albumin either as a manifestation of a poor nutritional state or as a result of a loss of albumin into the lumen of the gastrointestinal tract caused by the primary pathology (protein-losing enteropathy). Sometimes these more florid manifestations of malabsorption are not apparent and the diagnosis is only established after investigation of non-specific abdominal complaints or anaemia.

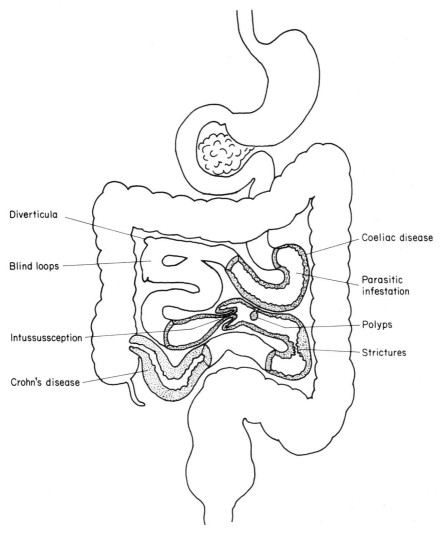

Fig. 4.3 *Important disorders of the small intestine.*

The diagnosis may be suspected as a result of a barium follow-through examination when dilated loops of small bowel will be identified with flocculation and segmentation of the barium. Malabsorption must then be confirmed by the assessment of the degree of steatorrhoea and the measurement of the malabsorption of various marker substances (see below). The specific cause of the malabsorption may become apparent during the course of radiological and absorptive function testing. Three major types of malabsorption can be identified.

(1) Disorders of digestion in which there is insufficient digestive enzymes or detergent effect within the small bowel. Since the intestinal mucosal cells are normal, the main feature of this type of malabsorption is steatorrhoea with deficiency of fat-soluble vitamins with little impairment of absorption of carbohydrate, protein, vitamin B_{12}, folate and iron.

(2) After gastric surgery, foodstuffs and digestive enzymes may never become adequately mixed thus resulting in another type of malabsorption. Furthermore, an extensive partial gastrectomy may result in inadequate production of intrinsic factor which is produced by parietal cells and is essential for the absorption of vitamin B_{12}. Without intrinsic factor, malabsorption of vitamin B_{12} alone is bound to occur.

(3) In chronic disorders of the pancreas, such as chronic pancreatitis, cystic fibrosis and pancreatic carcinoma, pancreatic enzymes are not produced in sufficient quantity to assist digestion of intraluminal contents and malabsorption may occur.

In recent years, it has been shown that an adequate concentration of bile salts within the intestinal lumen is essential for satisfactory absorption of fats and fat-soluble vitamins. This may occur when there has been surgical resection or disease involvement of the terminal ileum, since only here can bile salts be reabsorbed. Alternatively, in certain disorders, the upper small bowel may become colonized by undesirable bacteria which possess the ability to break down bile salts and render them unsuitable for their task of aiding fat and fat-soluble vitamin absorption. Some of these bacteria are also able to utilize vitamin B_{12} so that it is unavailable for absorption. This leads to anaemia secondary to vitamin B_{12} deficiency.

In other disorders causing malabsorption the intraluminal digestive phase is normal, but the absorptive cells are defective. This may be due to generalized mucosal damage from coeliac disease, tropical sprue, parasitic infestation or mucosal infiltration with disorders such as Crohn's disease or Whipple's disease. In these conditions, generalized malabsorption, may be demonstrated and mucosal damage identified. Other disorders have a histologically normal mucosa but malabsorption of a specific substance may be caused by the absence of a particular enzyme from the mucosa. The commonest example of this type of malabsorption is lactase deficiency in the small intestinal mucosal cells. As a result, the disaccharide lactose cannot be broken down to be absorbed as the simple sugars glucose and galactose.

Very rarely, defective transport of absorbed substances from the mucosal cell to the bloodstream or lacteals may occur. This is due to blockage of the lymphatic system by malignant disorders, tuberculosis or in the rare disorder of primary lymphangiectasia which involves the mesenteric lymphatic system.

Principal disorders causing malabsorption

Coeliac disease is characterized by an abnormal small intestinal mucosa. The mucosal damage is induced by gliadin, a component of the gluten protein of cereals. The exact mechanism of injury is uncertain but is probably due to local immunological responses. The normal small intestinal mucosa has numerous finger-like projections called villi which can be seen under the dissecting microscope or on histological section. In coeliac disease the villi become progressively shorter and eventually disappear resulting in a flat mucosa or 'subtotal villous atrophy'. As a result the absorptive surface area of the small intestine is greatly reduced and malabsorption will occur. Furthermore, since the epithelial cells of the villi produce digestive enzymes, defective intraluminal digestion will also be apparent (Fig. 4.4).

Coeliac disease usually begins in infancy when the child fails to thrive and may demonstrate voluminous pale stools with resulting growth retardation, anaemia and abdominal distension. On the other hand, the disorder may manifest in adult life when a spectrum of symptoms can occur varying from mild anaemia to florid malabsorption characterized by diarrhoea, weight loss and anaemia, peripheral neuropathy, osteomalacia and low serum albumin. As a late complication, sufferers with adult coeliac disease may develop malignant disease such as abdominal lymphoma or carcinoma.

The commonest cause of malabsorption in the world results from a reduction or absence of the disaccharidase enzyme lactase in the small intestinal mucosa. This occurs with a greater frequency than the normal population in patients with inflammatory bowel disease or those of Asian or African ethnic derivation. The commonest complaint is of vague abdominal discomfort with intermittent diarrhoea and colic. Reduction or elimination of lactose in the diet will usually improve symptoms. Very rarely, similar symptoms may be produced by mucosal deficiency of the disaccharidase enzymes which split fructose (fructase) or sucrose (sucrase).

Colonization of the proximal small bowel by abnormal bacteria may cause steatorrhoea, or anaemia due to vitamin B_{12} deficiency. Radiological investigation usually shows a lesion causing stasis in the intestine such as jejunal

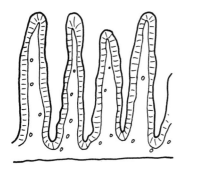
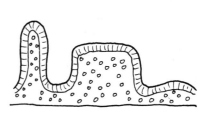

(a)   (b)

Fig. 4.4   Small intestinal villous structure. (a) Normal finger-like villi and (b) pathological villi, showing reduced height, broadening and increased round-cell infiltrate.

diverticula, previous gastric surgery, Crohn's disease, stricture formation in the small bowel or a fistulous communication between colon and small intestine. The diagnosis may be confirmed by identifying the presence of abnormal bacteria by the culture of jejunal aspirate, the deconjugation of bile salts in the proximal small bowel by breath tests, or alternative methods such as the measurement of urinary indican or the correction of streatorrhoea by a short course of antibiotics such as tetracycline. Although surgical correction of the identifiable cause of the contaminated small bowel syndrome is sometimes feasible, patients may often be rendered symptom-free by intermittent courses of antibiotics and supplementary vitamin B_{12} injections.

Crohn's disease is characterized by localized areas of non-specific granulomatous inflammation of the bowel. The alimentary tract may be affected anywhere from the mouth to the anus although the terminal ileum alone or terminal ileum and large bowel combined are most commonly involved. The disease may occur at any age but most commonly affects patients between the ages of 20 and 40 years, affecting both sexes equally. Whilst many patients can lead a reasonably normal life when the disease is active, in its chronic form it is an extremely debilitating condition which interferes greatly with the patient's life and causes repeated admissions to hospital for treatment.

The aetiology of Crohn's disease is unknown. Viruses and bacteria have been incriminated but no specific organisms have ever been isolated from intestinal contents, bowel wall or regional lymph nodes, all of which may be affected. It is currently believed that Crohn's disease is the result of a disturbed immune response in the gut wall, although the antigen has yet to be identified. Since Crohn's disease, ankylosing spondylitis and ulcerative colitis can all occur with increased frequency within family groups, it is suggested that all three diseases share a genetic basis. Macroscopically, the involved bowel is engorged and oedematous such that the lumen is markedly narrowed, sometimes enough to produce intestinal obstruction. The mucosa is oedematous and carries surface irregularities called 'cobble-stoning' with linear ulceration and fissures. The involvement is patchy within the gut and areas of normal bowel can be readily identified between the involved segments or 'skip' lesions. The affected lymph nodes and mesentery are also enlarged and thickened. Fistulae may develop between adjacent loops of bowel or between affected segments of bowel and bladder, uterus or vagina. Chronic perianal disease is common. Under the microscope, features are oedema and chronic inflammation with granulomas appearing in about half the cases.

Clinical features vary from case to case and depend largely upon the site and extent of bowel affected. In the acute form of the disease, acute appendicitis may be mimicked. In more chronic forms, abdominal pain and diarrhoea are the commonest symptoms, whilst an abdominal mass is frequently palpable. Malabsorption in Crohn's disease may be due to interference with bile salt reabsorption, colonization of the small bowel with abnormal bacteria, or direct involvement of the absorptive surfaces of the small bowel. Strictures and fistulae may promote abnormal bacterial colonization of the small intestine or lead to short circuits within the bowel, bypassing much of the absorptive surface area. In its chronic form, the disease is characterized by weight loss, low grade fever and moderate anaemia.

Radiology of the small and large bowel is the commonest method of identifying features suggestive of Crohn's disease, since the involved segments will be identified. Sometimes, a surgically resected segment is required to confirm the characteristic histological features. Most commonly, no conclusive proof of Crohn's disease is obtained and the diagnosis can only be presumptive, based on the nature of the radiological abnormality and the presence of various features of malabsorption.

Other diseases of the small intestine

Meckel's diverticulum is a congenital abnormality of the distal ileum. It is a little blind sac which occurs up to 60 cm from the ileocaecal valve and is usually about 5 cm long. Its major significance lies in a tendency to bleed either chronically or acutely. The acute bleeding episodes may be life-threatening. The presence of this congenital abnormality may be detected either by radiology or by ^{99m}technetium scanning.

Infection with the flagellate parasite *Giardia lambia* is worldwide but most common in the tropics. Its importance lies in the fact that the parasites attach to the duodenal and jejunal mucosa causing inflammation, partial villous atrophy and malabsorption. Recurrent attacks of abdominal pain, diarrhoea and steatorrhoea are characteristic. Giardiasis is diagnosed by recognizing cysts in the stools or the flagellate form in jejunal juice or mucus, or by identifying the parasite attached to the mucosa in a jejunal biopsy specimen.

Various tapeworms, roundworms and hookworms may infest the bowel leading to symptoms of abdominal discomfort and diarrhoea. Whilst not a major cause of malabsorption, long-term infestation may lead to anaemia, caused by iron or vitamin B_{12} deficiency. These disorders are diagnosed by detection of parasites or ova in stool specimens.

Infection of the gastrointestinal tract with a variety of bacteria and viruses most commonly leads to acute, severe, short term diarrhoea. It is rare for there to be any lasting effect on the small bowel mucosa although prolonged lactose intolerance or persistent diarrhoea may occasionally occur. In children, these acute diarrhoeal episodes may be particularly severe and may lead to dehydration and collapse. In Eastern countries, the most severe features of this type of illness are caused by infection of the gastrointestinal tract by the organism which causes cholera (*Vibrium cholerae*). In this severe disorder, large volumes of fluid gush effortlessly from stomach and bowel and severe dehydration may be evident within hours. Unless fluid and electrolytes are replaced, the patient may die as a result. Treatment lies in correcting electrolyte and fluid losses either by nasogastric tube or by rapid intravenous infusion, until the acute toxic effects are passed.

INVESTIGATIONS OF THE SMALL INTESTINE

Laboratory based tests:
  Lactose tolerance test
  Xylose absorption test
  Folic acid absorption studies
  Vitamin B_{12} absorption test
  Faecal fat analysis
  Stool analyses
Radiology:
  Barium follow-through
       small bowel enema
Gastroenterology department procedures:
  Jejunal biopsy
  Breath tests

Laboratory based

A routine inspection of a peripheral blood film by the Haematology laboratory may indicate the presence of anaemia. In malabsorption and small intestinal disease, anaemia may be iron deficient due either to bleeding into the small bowel or failure to absorb iron from the diet. The peripheral blood film may also show macrocytosis which may be due to impaired absorption of folic acid or vitamin B_{12}, or overutilization of vitamin B_{12} by bacteria in the contaminated small bowel syndrome. Biochemical analysis of peripheral blood may reveal hypoalbuminaemia due to malnutrition, or excessive protein loss from the small intestinal mucosal surface. A raised alkaline phosphatase may be an indication of bone disease secondary to malabsorption of vitamin D. Low serum cholesterol levels may also be present in malnutrition.

The absorption of various products of digestion take place at different levels in the small intestine. The major part of absorption takes place in the jejunum, where electrolytes, water, monosaccharides, amino acids and fats are absorbed. The only exceptions are vitamin B_{12} which is absorbed in the terminal ileum in the same area as the reabsorption of bile salts. Various tests have been elaborated to evaluate the adequacy of absorption of marker substances in order to assess the possibility of malabsorption. Test substances may be administered intravenously or orally and samples of blood, faeces, urine or even exhaled breath may be collected to assess small intestinal function (Fig. 4.5). Carbohydrate absorption may be evaluated using a lactose tolerance test. Normally, this disaccharide is broken down by intestinal lactase to the two monosaccharides glucose and galactose which are then absorbed. Should the enzyme lactase be deficient in the intestinal mucosa, a poor rise in blood glucose is seen and the patient may complain of colic and diarrhoea because the unabsorbed

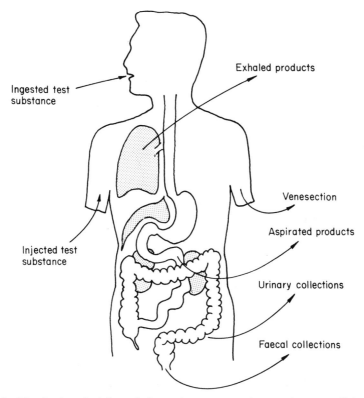

Ingested test substance

Exhaled products

Injected test substance

Venesection

Aspirated products

Urinary collections

Faecal collections

Fig. 4.5 *The basic principles of absorption tests used to evaluate small intestinal function.*

lactose acts as an osmotic agent in the gut. A similar test using sucrose or fructose may be used to assess the possibility that the small intestinal mucosa is deficient in the disaccharidases sucrase or fructase. The handling of carbohydrate by the small bowel may also be assessed in the xylose absorption test where 25 g of D-xylose is given orally after an overnight fast. Only a small proportion of the test substance is metabolized in the body and under normal circumstances 5–8 g should be excreted in the urine in a five-hour collection. Xylose absorption may be more accurately assessed by measuring a one-hour blood xylose level.

Fat excretion in the stools is a good assessment of the adequacy of fat absorption by the small intestine and faecal fat content may be measured by the laboratory after a three-day stool collection. Since the fat-soluble vitamins A, D and K are absorbed in the same way as dietary fat, measurement of the plasma vitamin A level is a useful indirect assessment of the adequacy of fat absorption.

Hydrolysis of dietary protein molecules is performed by gastric pepsin and pancreatic trypsin. Further hydrolysis takes place in the small intestine until a mixture of peptides and amino acids is absorbed into the small intestinal cells. Measurement of stool nitrogen provides a very crude assessment of the adequacy of dietary protein digestion, whilst excessive loss of albumin into the small bowel lumen can be measured by labelling albumin with radioactive chromium and measuring stool radioactivity over a three-day collection.

In the presence of anaemia, serum iron, serum folate and vitamin B_{12} levels may be measured by laboratory analysis of serum. Absorption of these substances may be tested using radioactively labelled test substances with subsequent measurement of serum radioactivity. The most commonly used test of this nature is the vitamin B_{12} absorption test in which the isotope may be administered without intrinsic factor and later with intrinsic factor to identify the possibility of pernicious anaemia due to intrinsic factor deficiency.

Stool microscopy is a valuable adjunct to the investigation of small bowel disease since microscopy may reveal the presence of parasites in the active or encysted forms, whilst stool culture may identify various pathogens (Fig. 4.5).

Radiology

A plain abdominal radiograph may identify distended small bowel loops, intestinal obstruction or gaseous distension in small bowel diverticula. A barium follow-through examination gives valuable information on the structure of the small bowel and the possible presence of strictures, fistulae or diverticula. A small bowel enema gives greater mucosal detail. Rarely, coeliac axis angiography may be performed where it is suspected that the arterial supply to the small intestinal arcades is in jeopardy causing small intestinal ischaemia.

Gastroenterology department based investigations

A jejunal biopsy is a technique used to obtain tissue from the mucosal surface of the small intestine for histological evaluation. The tiny mucosal biopsies may also be used to analyse the disaccharidase content of the mucosa. In these techniques, the mucosal specimen is obtained by asking the patient to swallow a capsule which is then negotiated into position in the small intestine under radiological control. When the capsule is positioned at the duodenojejunal flexure, specimens may be obtained. A variety of biopsy capsules are available for this technique. The most commonly used capsules, the Crosby and Watson capsules, have a spring-loaded blade which may be fired by external aspiration. The Cooke capsule contains no moving blade. The Medi-Tech biopsy system has a steerable capsule which may be negotiated into position more quickly and whose blade cuts the specimen by pulling on an external wire attached to the blade. Even more sophisticated is the Quinton–Reubin hydraulic capsule, in which the biopsy is cut by a hydraulically-operated blade which may be reloaded by hydraulic pressure. The biopsies obtained by this mechanism may be delivered externally without removing the tube and multiple biopsies may be obtained in similar fashion. This capsule is most commonly used in research work. Once obtained, the jejunal biopsy may be inspected under a dissecting microscope to assess the quality of the small intestinal villi, before being dispatched to the histological laboratory for microscopical analysis.

Analysis of exhaled breath has become valuable in the investigation of certain small intestinal disorders. After the administration of ^{14}C labelled bile salts, radioactive breath carbon dioxide may be collected. The amount of radioactivity within the breath, gives a direct indication of the rapidity of breakdown of the labelled bile salts within the small intestine. Rapid destruction of bile salts occurs when the small intestine is overgrown by pathological bacteria. Alternatively, the measurement of exhaled breath hydrogen may be undertaken. Hydrogen is one of the gases produced in the intestinal lumen by bacterial breakdown of carbohydrates and there appears to be a direct correlation between breath hydrogen excretion and hydrogen production in the intestinal lumen. As a result, breath hydrogen estimation may be used to measure carbohydrate malabsorption, excessive carbohydrate breakdown and abnormalities of small intestinal transit time. Earlier techniques to measure breath hydrogen were bedevilled by expensive and sophisticated equipment. More recently, simpler, cheaper instruments have become available which greatly facilitate its measurement. The major advantage of breath hydrogen tests over ^{14}C labelling techniques is that no isotope need be administered to the patient. The breath hydrogen tests are therefore of particular value in paediatric practice.

NURSING CARE DURING INVESTIGATION

Jejunal biopsies − capsule method (Fig. 4.6)

Check list

Capsule of choice: Crosby
                    Watson
                    Cooke
  Local anaesthetic spray
  Glass of water for patient
  Introducer wire
  Adhesive tape
  50 ml syringe
  Container for specimen
  2 ml syringe
  Needle
  Alcohol wipes

continued

Gauze swabs
Drugs: sedation
        metoclopramide
Dissecting microscope
Histology request form

Procedure

The capsule is assembled ready for use before the patient arrives after an overnight fast. The procedure is explained to the patient, reassurance is given and informed written consent obtained by the referring clinician. The 10-day rule should be observed if appropriate. Dentures are removed and the patient seated in a comfortable, upright chair.

The capsule is passed according to the method of choice. Local anaesthetic may help as may an introducer wire passed down the tube to facilitate the passage of the capsule over the tongue. Small sips of water may be given to help the patient swallow. Approximately 45 cm of the attached tubing should be swallowed whilst the patient is seated. If possible, the patient may now walk around for a few minutes before being positioned comfortably on a bed or trolley in the left lateral position. Metoclopramide 10 mg may be given intravenously or intramuscularly. Thirty centimetres more of tubing should be swallowed slowly without upsetting the patient. This position is maintained for twenty minutes.

The patient should now lie supine for twenty minutes with the feet elevated. The patient should then be positioned in the right lateral position with the bed or trolley returned to the horizontal. It is essential to use radiology to ascertain the correct position of the capsule. This can either be by a plain abdominal

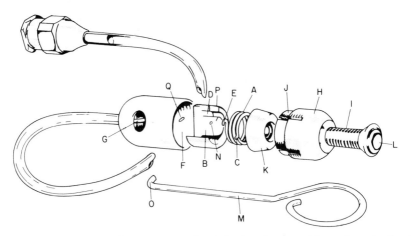

Fig. 4.6 *Watson Intestinal Biopsy Capsule. A, Spring; B, central boss; C, spring hook; D, slot; E, spring loop; F, open end of body; G, stake; H, cap; I, allen screw; J, skirt; K, collar; L, port in screw; M, loading rod; N, hole in knife; O, prong; P, groove; Q, stake.*

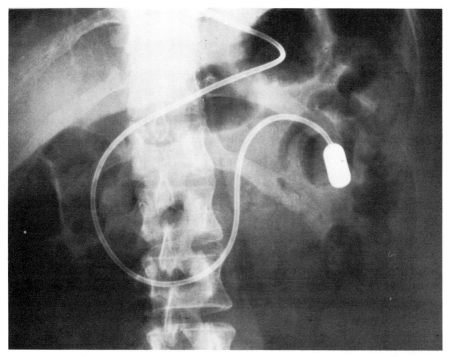

Fig. 4.7 *Jejunal biopsy capsule showing correct position pre-biopsy.*

radiograph or screening (Fig. 4.7). If the capsule is in the jejunum, a specimen may be obtained by attaching the 50 ml syringe to the capsule and 'firing' the blade by aspiration on the syringe which creates a vacuum within the capsule. The capsule should then be withdrawn by gentle pulling on the tube. If using a Cooke fixed-blade capsule, steady suction with the syringe should be maintained whilst a quick tug on the tube removes the biopsy specimen from the intestinal wall.

Once the specimen has been obtained, it may be inspected under the dissecting microscope or transferred directly to the Histopathology laboratory. Correct orientation of the biopsy specimen, with mucosal surface uppermost on a flat card, will be beneficial in obtaining a more reliable histological report. The patient should be made comfortable and may resume normal eating and drinking.

Jejunal biopsies – alternative techniques

Muzzle-loading via the endoscope (Fig. 4.8)

Check list

As for routine upper gastrointestinal endoscopy, with the addition of a capsule of choice adapted by having a longer length of tubing attached. This tubing is then threaded back through the biopsy channel of the endoscope and a reasonable length of tubing is left protruding from the proximal end of the biopsy channel.

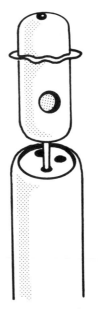

Fig. 4.8 *'Muzzle-loaded' jejunal biopsy capsule protruding from tip of end-viewing gastroscope.*

Procedure

The capsule is held in position close to the distal tip of the instrument and within vision during endoscopy, and the endoscope is steered by the normal method into the duodenum.

The tubing is then fed down the channel and when the capsule is in the correct position a specimen may be obtained, as described above. Radiology is not necessary for this technique.

Steerable system (Fig. 4.9)

A steerable biopsy system may be used to guarantee a jejunal biopsy rapidly.

Check list

Steerable catheter biopsy system assembled according to the manufacturer's instructions
Local anaesthetic spray
Lubrication
Drugs: diazepam
        metoclopramide
Radiological contrast medium

continued

Syringes: 10 ml for vacuum purposes
         20 ml for contrast medium
         2 ml for drugs
Alcohol wipes
Gauze swabs
Adhesive tape

Procedure

The patient arrives after an overnight fast, when the procedure is explained, reassurance given and informed written consent obtained by the referring clinician. The 10-day rule should be observed if appropriate. Dentures are removed and the patient positioned in the left lateral position on the screening table. Local anaesthetic may be applied to the throat. Sedation and metoclopramide may be given intravenously if required. A mouth guard must be used if the patient has teeth.

The catheter is lubricated and steered into place under radiological control. Contrast may be introduced via the catheter to help outline the gastrointestinal tract, but this should be rinsed away with plain water and air passed through the catheter before any attempt is made to obtain the specimen. When the tip of the catheter is at the duodenojejunal junction, the pressure gauge is fixed to the controls, the syringe applied to obtain a vacuum, and the wire pulled to obtain

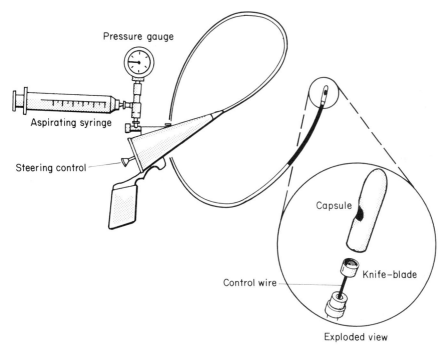

Fig. 4.9 *Meditech steerable jejunal biopsy system.*

the specimen. The catheter is withdrawn and the biopsy removed. If required, more specimens may now be obtained by repeating the above procedure. When the procedure is complete, the patient is allowed to recover as from routine endoscopy and may resume normal eating and drinking. The local anaesthetic, sedation and metoclopramide are not essential and may be omitted. The biopsy specimen should be transported promptly to the Histopathology laboratory with the completed request form.

Complications of jejunal biopsy

These are usually mechanical problems due to either the failure of the capsule to fire or disintegration of the capsule while in use. If the capsule is lost in the gastrointestinal tract it will pass naturally; progress may be observed with fluoroscopy if necessary. Should it be difficult to remove the capsule at the end of the procedure, sedation may be given to relax the patient. Perforation is rare; routine care for acute abdominal illness will be required should this occur.

Complications of the steerable system are as for routine OGD.

^{14}C glycine cholic acid breath test (Fig. 4.10)

Check list

Tray with glass of cold milk and slice of bread and butter or Lundh meal (see Lundh test, p. 179)
Collection equipment for expired air:
  Glass syringe − the barrel only of a 20 ml syringe
  Gauze
  Cork
  Glass tubing
  Aspirating needle
Drying agent: fused granular calcium chloride
Indicator: Thymolphthalein 0.2% in scintillation fluid in four containers provided by the Isotope laboratory
Isotope: 5 μci ^{14}C-labelled glycine cholic acid in ethanol to be added to the milk or Lundh meal
The 10-day rule does not apply to this isotope

Procedure

The patient arrives after an overnight fast. The procedure is explained, the patient reassured and consent obtained by the referring clinician. The isotope is added to the test meal. The patient is weighed and the weight recorded. The meal is now administered.

The patient is allowed to sit quietly in a comfortable chair and discouraged from any activity. Expired air is collected at hourly intervals for four hours by the patient breathing normally to the end of vital capacity, then blowing expired air over the drying agent. This takes 2–3 minutes. The specimens are sent to the laboratory labelled and with a completed request form. The patient may then eat and drink normally.

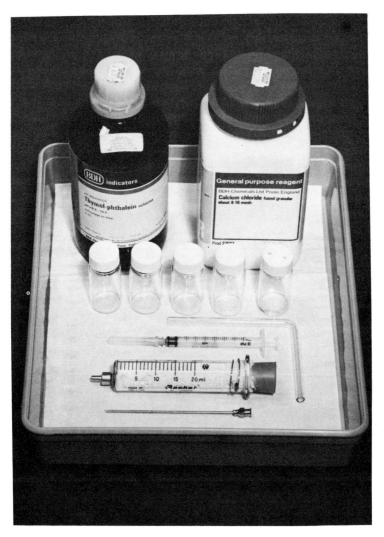

Fig. 4.10 *Equipment for ^{14}C glycine cholic acid breath test.*

5

THE HEPATOBILIARY SYSTEM

THE LIVER

Anatomy

The liver is the largest organ in the body, weighing 1200–1500 g. It is vital for life since it is the only site of important metabolic functions. It is reddish-brown in colour and is situated in the right upper quadrant of the abdomen just below the diaphragm. It has two lobes; a larger right and a small left lobe separated by a fibrous ligament anteriorly and posteriorly. It is somewhat irregular in shape. The superior surface is in contact with the under-surface of the right side of the diaphragm, which separates it from the base of the right lung. The inferior surface is closely related to the other abdominal viscera including the right kidney, the colon and the stomach on the left. The anterior surface of the liver is separated from the right lower ribs and costal cartilages by the diaphragm laterally, whilst anteriorly it is closely related to the anterior abdominal wall. The posterior surface crosses the vertebral column in the mid-line and lies in close relationship to the aorta, inferior vena cava and cardio–oesophageal junction. In the centre of the inferior surface is the hilum through which enters the hepatic artery and portal vein and at which site the main bile ducts leave the liver. The gall bladder is attached to the inferior surface of the right lobe. The liver is covered by a fibrous capsule and in the greater part, by a layer of peritoneum.

The organ is built up of a large number of lobules. The liver cells are organized into regular columns and separated by spaces called sinusoids. Between the lobules are supporting structures called portal tracts which contain branches of the hepatic artery, the portal vein, lymphatics and bile ducts. Each lobule receives a blood supply from branches of the hepatic artery and portal vein via the portal tracts and the blood filters through each lobule into a central vein which is a tributary of the hepatic vein. Bile is produced in the sinusoids and passes to small bile ducts in the portal tract. These gradually unite to form the main right and left intrahepatic bile ducts.

A double set of blood vessels supplying blood to the liver make the organ unique. Blood is brought by the hepatic artery which is a branch of the coeliac axis coming from the abdominal aorta. This conveys oxygenated blood which nourishes the liver cells and supplies them with oxygen necessary for their vital functions. In addition, blood is brought to the liver by the portal vein which contains venous blood rich in absorbed foodstuffs from the intestine and also containing blood from the stomach and spleen. Through this vessel the liver receives the substrates vital for its metabolic function.

Blood leaves the liver via the hepatic vein which arises from the union of the many centrilobular veins and then drains into the inferior vena cava.

Physiology

The liver is concerned in the metabolism of the three principle foodstuffs, carbohydrate, protein and fat. It also secretes bile, manufactures serum proteins and clotting substances and stores vitamin B_{12} and iron. A number of drugs are altered in composition and toxic substances are destroyed by the action of liver cells.

Carbohydrate taken in the food is broken down by digestive juices and absorbed by the small intestine. It reaches the liver as glucose and fructose. These sugars may pass through the liver directly to the blood stream or alternatively converted to a storage carbohydrate called glycogen. Glycogen may be reconverted into glucose according to the body's need for sugar for metabolic requirements. This function of the liver is controlled by the hormone insulin, secreted by the pancreas and by adrenalin circulating in the bloodstream.

The end products of protein digestion are the amino acids which are brought to the liver via the portal vein. In the liver, the nitrogen present in the excess amino acid is converted into a breakdown substance called urea which is carried by the bloodstream from the liver to the kidneys where it is excreted in the urine. The retained amino acids are the important constituents of the structures and tissues of all organs of the body. Wear and tear within these structures is continually made good by repair processes using the amino acids supplied by the liver. The important plasma proteins, albumin and globulin, are synthesized from amino acids by the liver.

Fat reaches the liver in the form of fatty acids. They may be conveyed to the fat stores of the body where they are stored as saturated fats and they must be desaturated by recycling through the liver before being available as an energy source for the tissues of the body (Fig. 5.1).

Secretion of bile

Bile is formed by the liver cells and is secreted into the canaliculi between the columns of liver cells. These empty into the bile ducts within the portal tracts which gradually join to form the right and left intrahepatic ducts. These join to form the common hepatic duct just outside the liver. The bile formed in this

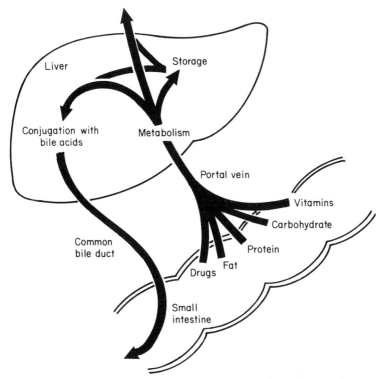

Fig. 5.1   *Liver metabolism of substances absorbed from the small intestine.*

way is stored in the gall bladder and subsequently passes down the common bile duct to be mixed with duodenal contents. Bile is alkaline in reaction and contains bile pigments, produced from haemoglobin after the breakdown of red blood cells, and bile acids which are produced in the liver from cholesterol. Small amounts of bile pigment (bilirubin) and the bile acids (cholic and cheno-deoxycholic acid) are reabsorbed in the terminal ileum and re-excreted by the liver. This enterohepatic circulation of bile constituents may occur many times a day and allows large amounts of bile acid to be delivered to the intestine daily from a relatively small total bile acid pool. It has been estimated that up to ten recyclings may occur each day (Fig. 5.2)

In the small intestine, bile acids combine with fatty acids to form micelles which increase the efficiency of fat absorption. Insufficiency of bile acids results in poor absorption of both fats and fat-soluble vitamins. Such a deficiency of bile acids may be caused by liver disease, biliary obstruction or small intestinal overgrowth of bacteria capable of deconjugating the bile acids. Interruption of the enterohepatic circulation by disease or resection of the terminal ileum leads to excessive bile acids in the colon and a resultant unavailability for recirculation. This too, leads to a deficiency of bile acids in the small intestine.

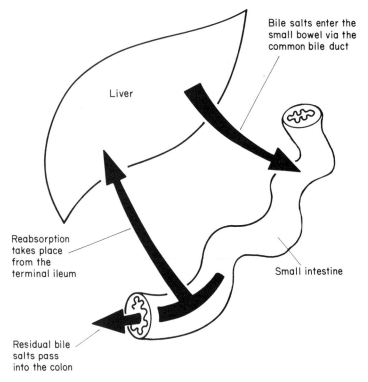

Fig. 5.2   *The enterohepatic circulation of bile salts.*

Under these circumstances, the bile acids in the colon act as an irritant and cause watery diarrhoea.

Vitamin and hormone metabolism

The liver has an important role in the storage of some vitamins. These include vitamin A, D, K, B_{12} and folic acid. In addition to the storage of the vitamins, vitamin D and folic acid are converted to more active forms while vitamin K is used by the liver cells for the production of coagulation factors.

Many hormones are metabolized and inactivated by the liver. These include thyroxin, antidiuretic hormones and steroid hormones such as cortisol and oestrogens. Failure to inactivate some of these hormones during liver cell failure contributes to the features manifest during that clinical condition, such as fluid retention and breast enlargement in men.

Drug metabolism

The liver is the most important organ for drug metabolism in the body. Most drugs metabolized are fat soluble and in the liver they are converted into water soluble substances making them suitable for excretion in bile or urine. Two types of reaction occur; first oxidation, reduction or hydroxylation reactions and secondly, conjugation reactions, to produce bile soluble substances. The liver metabolizes about 90% of alcohol ingested. The enzyme system responsible for this reaction is capable of being induced or made more vigorous by repeated alcoholic ingestion. Since the enzyme system also metabolizes certain drugs, habitual drinkers may be resistant to the action of such drugs. In addition, in liver disease, drug metabolism may be impaired and care is needed to avoid overdosage particularly with sedative drugs. This may be important during sedation for endoscopy and other gastrointestinal procedures.

Immunological function

Approximately 20% of the liver cell mass is comprised of reticuloendothelial cells. These cells have important but poorly understood immunological functions by destroying foreign protein absorbed from the gut, removing immune complexes from the blood and by removing dying constituents from the bloodstream. It is possible, but not yet proven, that the liver is also the site of important antibody production.

Pathology

Hepatitis

Inflammation of the liver is called hepatitis and its most common cause is a virus infection. Such infections are characterized by general malaise, fever and jaundice with intolerance to fats. The episode is most commonly of acute onset and of short duration. During the attack, liver function tests are abnormal but gradually return to basal levels. Most commonly, viral hepatitis is caused by hepatitis A virus and all traces of virus particles which might cause infectivity have passed from the patient before jaundice occurs. On the other hand, the more severe type of infective hepatitis caused by hepatitis B virus is a more serious condition, since virus particles may be identified within the bloodstream long after the initial episode so that the patients remain infective. In many cases of hepatitis of this nature, serum studies are unable to detect evidence of hepatitis A or hepatitis B virus and it is now known that other viruses called 'non-A, non-B' hepatitis virus also exist.

The persistent infectivity of some patients who have had hepatitis B virus infection is of major importance to hospital workers since that patient's blood may be capable of transmitting infection to anyone in contact with it. Such persistent infectivity is most common in drug addicts, homosexuals and residents of long-stay hospitals, particularly mental institutions. Hospital departments where blood or plasma products are in high usage are also important areas. These include blood transfusion units, transplant units and renal dialysis units. Contact with patients' blood and body fluids is also common in gastrointestinal procedures, where similar precautions are important. It is now standard practice for blood donors, transplant patients and dialysis patients to have been screened for the presence of virus particles of hepatitis B in their blood. Doctors and nurses working with hepatitis B positive patients must avoid contact with the patient's blood and must always wear gloves during procedures. Should contact with blood or blood products from such a patient occur, then gammaglobulin injections are available to protect the worker from an acute attack. A vaccine against hepatitis B is now available. It will be of value for all hospital workers in 'at risk' situations.

Chronic active hepatitis

Chronic active hepatitis is a condition in which the liver function tests reflect continuing liver cell damage, whilst the patient may suffer a varying degree of illness from being asymptomatic, through vague malaise and lassitude to overt jaundice and signs of liver failure. Most commonly, immunological studies suggest an immune basis for the condition with the presence of smooth muscle antibodies. However, the condition may also be produced after viral hepatitis, with certain drugs such as methyldopa, as a result of excessive alcoholic consumption and during the course of Wilson's disease. Histologically, the condition is characterized by destruction of liver cells in a continuous low-grade process. In more severe cases, so called chronic aggressive hepatitis, large sheets of liver cells may be killed simultaneously and pockets of necrosis of liver cells may bridge from the centrilobular vein to the portal tract. This degree of histological abnormality carries a more severe prognosis. Immunosuppressive therapy is of value in controlling the liver cell damage.

Primary biliary cirrhosis, a condition in which the immunological insult is directed to the small bile canaliculi, may be confused with chronic active hepatitis but can usually be distinguished by different immunological studies and liver biopsy features. Primary biliary cirrhosis is more common in females than in males and has a slowly progressive and insidious downhill course. No specific treatment is yet available although recent studies with D-penicillamine are hopeful.

Cirrhosis of the liver

Cirrhosis is characterized by hardening, nodularity and enlargement of the liver. These features are produced by the mixture of necrosis of liver cells, nodular regeneration and distortion of the liver architecture by fibrous septa. Micronodular cirrhosis is characterized by regular septa with regenerative nodules approximate in size to the original lobules, whilst macronodular cirrhosis is characterised by fibrous septa of varying thickness with marked difference in size of the regenerative nodules. In mixed cirrhosis, features of both types of fibrosis may be identified. In many cases, the aetiology of cirrhosis is difficult to identify and the prime cause varies geographically. In Britain, cirrhosis is usually associated with alcohol abuse, chronic active hepatitis or primary biliary cirrhosis. Rarer causes of cirrhosis include haemochromatosis,

Wilson's disease, glycogen storage disease, drug therapy with methyldopa, secondary cholestasis or venous congestion as seen in hepatic vein thrombosis or chronic heart failure. In many cases, no single cause for the cirrhosis can be detected. Under these circumstances, the cirrhosis is said to be cryptogenic in origin. Manifestations of cirrhosis are variable and it is certainly true that patients can be asymptomatic with quite severe degrees of liver disturbance. The patient may complain of weakness, fatigue, weight loss or vague dyspeptic symptoms. Otherwise, clinical features are due mainly to the presence of portal hypertension or hepatic insufficiency.

Portal hypertension results from destruction and distortion of the veins running through the liver thus forcing the blood back into the portal vein and its tributaries. As a result, the blood must find an alternative route to the heart and collateral circulations are set up in various sites, the most common of which is in the lower oesophagus. As more blood flows through these collaterals, they become distended and tortuous and are called oesophageal varices. Alternative sites for such collateral circulations are around the umbilicus or in the rectum. The commonest complication of oesophageal varices is profuse haemorrhage into the gastrointestinal tract. For this, balloon tamponade with a Sengstaken–Blakemore tube, endoscopic sclerotherapy, oesophageal transection or even portacaval shunt surgery may become necessary (Fig. 5.3).

The spleen usually becomes enlarged as part of the process of portal hypertension, although it is seldom greatly enlarged. When the spleen is not enlarged, portal hypertension is unlikely. Fluid may accumulate within the abdomen and this is called ascites. Although portal hypertension contributes to its formation, other factors such as endocrine disturbance and hypoalbuminaemia as part of the liver cell failure may also play a part. Jaundice is due mainly to failure of bilirubin metabolism whilst intrahepatic cholestasis may be a contributing factor. Jaundice is generally mild or absent and increasing jaundice implies progressive liver failure. A haemorrhagic tendency is often found in advanced liver disease and is due to poor production of coagulation factors by the damaged liver cells. A lowered platelet count as a result of splenomegaly, may also be contributory. Bruising, purpura, nose-bleeds or gastrointestinal haemorrhage can all result.

Mental disturbance during liver cells failure is known as hepatic encephalopathy. The earliest features are slight drowsiness with poor concentration, but may progress through behavioural abnormalities including aggressive outbursts and mania, to drowsiness and coma. Rarely, paraplegia, Parkinsonism, fits and dementia suggest more formal and focal brain damage. A number of factors may precipitate hepatic encephalopathy in cirrhotic patients. These include drugs, anaesthesia, a high protein diet, intercurrent infection, gastrointestinal bleeding, electrolyte disturbance and even constipation.

It is clear that cirrhosis may be variable in its presentation. Patients may be asymptomatic for many years but may eventually present with manifestations of liver cell failure such as a haemorrhagic tendency or ascites. The development

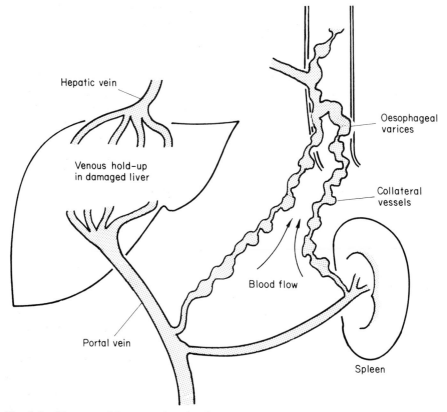

Fig. 5.3   *How portal hypertension develops.*

of portal hypertension may result in the presence of splenomegaly or bleeding from oesophageal varices. Much more sinister, is the development of hepatic encephalopathy by any one of the precipitants mentioned above.

In acute hepatic necrosis, developing anew or superimposed upon established cirrhosis, all of these features of hepatocellular failure may be manifest.

Alcohol and the liver

It is known that alcohol may damage the liver in a variety of ways. An acute alcoholic episode may produce a hepatitis-like event which will settle completely provided alcohol is withdrawn. Continuing alcohol abuse may produce fatty change in the liver or the features of chronic active hepatitis. Prolonged damage of this nature will eventually lead to the development of fibrous septa and nodular regeneration, the hallmarks of cirrhosis. It is important to identify that alcohol may be the cause of a particular patient's liver disease since the liver has the potential for total recovery provided fibrosis has not become superimposed. Total abstinence is the key to recovery and patients may be reassured that they have the potential to return to full health.

Cancer of the liver

The commonest cause of cancer of the liver is metastatic growth from a primary lesion in the gastrointestinal tract or lung. Alternatively, hepatoma may occur as a late complication of chronic alcoholism or chronic active hepatitis, especially if this state is produced in a chronic hepatitis B carrier. The incidence of primary hepatocellular cancer is very variable worldwide. Primary cancer arising within the liver from bile duct tissue (cholangiocarcinoma) is also very rare and usually slow growing. This latter form of cancer usually presents at a late stage with jaundice due to obstruction of the bile ducts at the porta hepatis.

GALL BLADDER AND BILE DUCTS

Anatomy and physiology (Fig. 5.4)

The smallest intrahepatic bile channels are formed in the lobules between the liver cells. The channels gradually unite with those of larger size to form the right and left hepatic ducts. These exit from the liver at the porta hepatis on the inferior surface, and join immediately to form the common hepatic duct. About 5 cm below the liver edge, the common hepatic duct is joined by the cystic duct from the gall bladder to form the common bile duct, which passes downwards behind the duodenum and then into the substance of the head of the pancreas. It emerges on the medial wall of the second part of the duodenum at the small papilla called the ampulla of Vater. In this area, it is usually joined by the pancreatic duct so that they have a common exit into the duodenum. The total length of the common bile duct varies from 2–9 cm.

The gall bladder is a small pear-shaped sac with a capacity of about 50 ml, situated under the right lobe of the liver. The cystic duct connects the gall bladder to the common bile duct. The wall of the gall bladder consists of an outer peritoneal coat continuous with the peritoneum generally, a muscular coat, contraction of which causes the gall bladder to empty into the common bile duct and an inner coat of mucous membrane which has the ability to absorb water from dilute bile within the gall bladder.

The liver secretes bile continuously and produces 1–2 l daily under a pressure of 15–25 cm H_2O. Since the resting pressure in the common bile duct is higher than that in the gall bladder, bile flows into the gall bladder where it is concentrated by water and electrolyte absorption. Gall bladder contraction is produced by cholecystokinin which is secreted by the duodenal mucosa in response to food. Contraction of the gall bladder causes concentrated bile to be injected into the common bile duct and thence into the second part of the duodenum

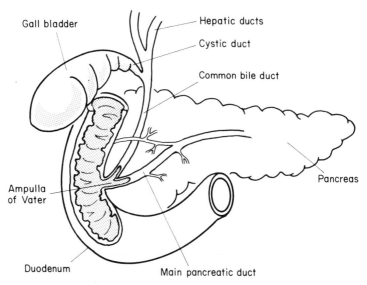

Fig. 5.4   *Anatomical relationships of the gall bladder and bile ducts.*

where it mixes with foodstuffs, aids in neutralization of acid gastric contents and facilitates fat absorption.

Pathology

Gallstones

Gallstone formation is the commonest disorder of the biliary tract and occurs when there is an excess of cholesterol in the bile with insufficient bile salts to keep it in solution. Evidence now suggests that abnormal bile of this nature must be present for a considerable time before gallstones are produced. Some gallstones are composed almost wholly of calcium salts or bilirubin, the latter occurring when there has been prolonged overproduction of bilirubin due to haemolysis of red blood cells. By far the commonest gallstones however, are those consisting mainly of cholesterol. Although the liver produces the abnormal bile, the gall bladder is the site of gallstone formation since it provides an area for cholesterol precipitation and a reservoir for gallstone growth. Previous infection and inflammation in the gall bladder may increase the tendency to form gallstones as may disease or removal of the terminal ileum, cirrhosis of the liver and long-term oral contraceptive therapy. Whilst gallstones are produced in the gall bladder they may migrate into the common bile duct where they can produce obstructive jaundice. Sometimes a gallstone may become impacted in the cystic duct. In this case, the gall bladder will be unable to empty and will become progressively more distended. The retained bile frequently becomes infected to produce a gall bladder full of pus. This condition is called empyema of the gall bladder. Recurrent attacks of acute inflammation of the gall bladder may be superimposed upon the presence of gallstones. This condition is called acute cholecystitis, and is characterized by more constant pain in the right upper quadrant of the abdomen associated with a high fever and high white blood cell count. Sometimes, the patient may experience severe colicky pain in the same area, which is caused by the passage of a stone down the cystic duct or the common bile duct and is called biliary colic.

By far the most common symptom complex of gall bladder disease is the presence of vague indigestion, upper abdominal discomfort with nausea and belching particularly after fatty foods. This state is called chronic cholecystitis and may or may not be accompanied by the presence of gallstones. A poorly functioning gall bladder is usually identified radiologically.

Sometimes, the bile ducts themselves are the site of pathology which may or may not be related to pathology within the gall bladder. Gallstones produced in the gall bladder may become impacted in the common bile duct where they may simply cause recurrent jaundice which may or may not be painful. Most commonly, the patient experiences recurrent attacks of biliary colic, jaundice and fever, the triad of symptoms known as ascending cholangitis. Gallstones retained within the common bile duct after surgery, commonly produce similar symptoms. Rarely, strictures of the common bile duct may be produced.

Sclerosing cholangitis is a rare condition in which the biliary system is gradually obliterated by fibrotic changes which probably has an immunological basis. It may be associated with ulcerative colitis, retroperitoneal fibrosis or secondary to the presence of gallstones. Progressive cholestasis and eventually secondary biliary cirrhosis are the usual outcome of the condition.

Carcinoma within the biliary system is very rare. Carcinoma of the gall bladder is usually an adenocarcinoma and presents typically with features similar to chronic cholecystitis. Indeed, the presence of gallstones is a common accompaniment, whilst calcification of the gall bladder is associated with cancer within its walls. Carcinoma of the bile ducts (cholangiocarcinoma) is an even more uncommon tumour which may arise anywhere in the biliary tree from the small intrahepatic bile ducts down to the ampulla of Vater. Obstructive jaundice is the usual presenting feature, although this may be delayed when the tumour is intrahepatic and involves only the right or left hepatic duct. Serum alphafetoprotein is never elevated under these circumstances, thus differentiating the condition from primary hepatocellular carcinoma. Cholangiocarcinoma has been described as a late complication in chronic ulcerative colitis.

INVESTIGATIONS OF THE HEPATOBILIARY SYSTEM

Venous blood tests:
  Liver function tests
  Serum virology studies
  Serum immunological studies

continued

Radiological and imaging techniques:
  Plain abdominal radiography
  Oral cholecystography and intravenous cholangiography with tomography
  Percutaneous transhepatic cholangiography and drainage
  Endoscopic retrograde cholangiography
  Trans-splenic portal venography
  Angiography
  Ultrasonography
  Isotopic liver scans
  CAT scans
Gastroenterology department procedures:
  Endoscopic retrograde cholangiopancreatography and nasobiliary drainage
  Liver biopsy
  Laparoscopy

Liver function tests

The term liver function tests refers to a group of biochemical investigations which are useful in confirming that the liver is diseased and indicating whether the liver cells or the biliary tract is primarily involved. The term is misleading since many of the investigations do not truly measure liver function but are useful indicators of the state of the liver. It is useful under this heading to consider also, various biochemical tests useful in detecting the cause of various diseases of the liver.

The following are useful tests.

Serum bilirubin

Jaundice is due to an elevated serum bilirubin which may be due to haemolysis, liver cell damage or obstruction to bile flow in the common bile duct. Bilirubin may be unconjugated or conjugated by its passage through the liver. Increase in the unconjugated fraction without any abnormalities of other liver function tests, usually results from haemolysis or from an inability to transport bilirubin across the liver cells. This latter state is called Gilbert's syndrome. Elevation of the conjugated fraction of serum bilirubin, indicates hepatobiliary disease and other tests of liver function are almost always abnormal. Bilirubin is usually present in the urine in addition. The highest concentrations of serum bilirubin occur most frequently in biliary tract obstruction and primary biliary cirrhosis. Sensitive and inexpensive dipstick tests for bilirubin in the urine are available and useful. The presence of bilirubin in the urine points to hepatobiliary disease. The absence of bilirubin in the urine of a jaundiced patient suggests haemolysis.

A simple dipstick test is also available to detect the presence of urobilinogen in the urine. Small amounts of urobilinogen are usually present especially in afternoon urine. Increased urinary urobilinogen occurs in haemolytic diseases but in these patients bilirubin is absent from the urine. Liver disease will result in increased urobilinogen in the urine whilst the total absence of urobilinogen in the urine for over a week indicates complete biliary obstruction.

Liver enzymes

Several enzymes appear in the blood as a result of liver cell damage. The most important of these are the transferases, known as aspartate transaminase (AST) (or glutamic oxaloacetic transaminase (GOT)) and alanine transferase (ALT) (or glutamic pyruvic transaminase). Irrespective of the cause, whenever liver cells are damaged or killed, these enzymes are liberated into the blood. Measurement of transferases is therefore a direct measure of the severity of acute liver damage.

Alkaline phosphatase occurs in almost all tissues, mainly bone and liver. When liver cells are damaged, little alkaline phosphatase is liberated into the blood, but when the biliary tract is obstructed at any level, extra alkaline phosphatase is synthesized in liver cell membranes and leaks into the blood. A greatly increased blood alkaline phosphatase level is therefore the main indicator of biliary obstruction. Sometimes an elevated serum alkaline phosphatase may be detected co-incidentally and when all other liver function tests are normal. The source of this alkaline phosphatase may be detected by electrophoretic separation of the various types of alkaline phosphatase from various sites. These various types of alkaline phosphatase are called isoenzymes.

Two other enzymes are of great importance since they are more specific to liver cells. These are 5-nucleotidase and gamma-glutamyl transpeptidase (gamma GT). Gamma GT is the most sensitive indicator of liver cell damage.

Plasma proteins

The liver is the only source of production of serum albumin. In chronic liver disease, serum albumin concentrations are frequently below normal, indicating impaired hepatic synthesis. Reduced serum albumin concentrations may contribute to the ascites and peripheral oedema in patients with cirrhosis. It is characteristic of chronic liver disease that elevated serum globulin also occurs. This hyperglobulinaemia represents a reaction of the reticuloendothelial system in general, and does not directly reflect liver cell damage. Indeed, the causes of hyperglobulinaemia are not fully understood, although they probably reflect an increase in activity of the immune system and suggest an immunological basis for the liver disease.

Coagulation factors

Severe liver cell damage impairs the production of prothrombin as well as other important coagulation factors produced by the liver. This is most readily detected by the one-stage prothrombin time which is a most sensitive index of liver cell damage. Prolongation of the prothrombin time may be found in severe acute hepatitis and in drug-induced liver damage. The prothrombin time is a valuable prognostic guide; an abnormal value indicates severe damage and increasing prothrombin time indicates a progressively worse prognosis. In suspected liver disease it is important to measure the prothrombin time prior to performing a liver biopsy.

Useful serum tests in liver disease

Serum alphafetoprotein when markedly elevated, is suggestive of hepatocellular carcinoma. Serum caeruloplasmin is a copper-containing globulin produced by the liver and is low or undetectable in Wilson's disease. A high serum iron with a highly saturated iron-binding capacity and elevated serum ferritin concentrations are diagnostic of haemochromotosis. Absence of alpha 1-antitrypsin enzyme from the serum is a marker of this deficiency which causes liver disease in infancy and childhood. It rarely causes cirrhosis in adults.

Serum virology studies

Hepatitis A infections are probably the commonest cause of jaundice around the world. The hepatitis A antigen (HAAg) is excreted in the stools during the last two weeks of the incubation period but then disappears at the onset of clinical illness. The antibody to hepatitis A virus (anti-HAV) appears in the blood at the onset of symptoms and is an important marker for diagnosis. The serum test for its performance is readily performed in virus laboratories.

Of far greater importance in the community at large and more especially to hospital staff involved in treatment with such patients, is infection with the hepatitis B virus. The hepatitis B virus contains several antigens to which infected persons can make immune responses. These antigens and their antibodies are important in identifying hepatitis B virus infection as the cause of jaundice and in recognizing a status of continuing infectivity in any one patient. The hepatitis B surface antigen (HBsAg) is located in the capsule of the virus. It can be identified by haemagglutination and radioimmunoassay methods and is a reliable marker of hepatitis B virus infection. It usually appears in the blood late in the incubation period or early in the onset of symptoms of acute type B hepatitis. It may be present for only a few days but usually lasts up to three months. Antibody to HBsAg (anti-HBs) usually appears after about three months and may persist for many years or even permanently. Its presence implies only that infection has occurred at some time. The central part of the virus contains an antigen called the core antigen (HBcAg) which is not found in the blood but which stimulates the production of an antibody (anti-HBc) which appears early in the disease and then only gradually subsides. This antibody is considered to be an index of infection and of viral replication. Its presence in the serum of patients who have suffered type B hepatitis indicates continuing infectivity and the risk that such patients may transmit the disease to workers who come into contact with their blood or blood-containing secretions. Persistence of the hepatitis B virus after acute type B hepatitis may lead to chronic hepatitis, cirrhosis or even hepatocellular carcinoma.

Other viruses which may cause jaundice and liver damage include cyto-megalovirus, Epstein–Barr virus and rubella virus. Serological tests for these viruses are all readily available to aid diagnosis.

Serum immunological studies

Three auto-antibodies in the blood are important in liver disease; antinuclear antibody, smooth muscle antibody and antimitochondrial antibody. None of these are specific to liver disease since antinuclear and antimitochondrial anti-bodies occur in connective tissue diseases and in other autoimmune diseases including thyroid disorders and pernicious anaemia. Equally, smooth muscle antibody has been reported in a variety of malignant diseases. In liver disease, smooth muscle antibody is usually elevated in chronic hepatitis whilst antimito-chondrial antibody is elevated in primary biliary cirrhosis. This distinction is used as an aid to differentiate these two chronic liver disorders. None of the autoantibodies actually damage liver tissue and they are unlikely to have signifi-cant aetiological importance.

Radiological and ultrasonography techniques

Conventional radiology

Many conventional radiological techniques can give valuable information with regard to liver, gall bladder and bile ducts. A plain abdominal radiograph may indicate air under the diaphragm, a fluid level in an abscess in the liver, air in the bile ducts or stones in the region of the gall bladder or biliary tree.

Oral cholecystography remains the most useful investigation for the assess-ment of gall bladder function and disease. A cholecystogram will usually demonstrate the ability of the gall bladder to concentrate dye, its ability to con-tract after a fatty meal and the presence or absence of gallstones. With the advent of gallstone dissolution therapy, these features of biliary disease take on added importance since dissolution therapy can only be contemplated and its progress monitored if the gall bladder is functioning, the stones are less than 1 cm in diameter and are radiolucent. The technique depends upon the patient taking tablets of a radio-opaque iodine-containing dye by mouth in the 24 hours prior to the procedure. Subsequently, the patient attends the Radiology depart-ment and plain abdominal films assess the concentration of the dye by the gall bladder. A fatty meal is then administered by mouth and one hour later further abdominal films are taken to see whether the gall bladder has contracted.

Intravenous cholangiography has, for many years, been the only method of identifying stones in the common bile duct. Its application has been limited by poor definition in the jaundiced patient and by allergic reactions to the dye in

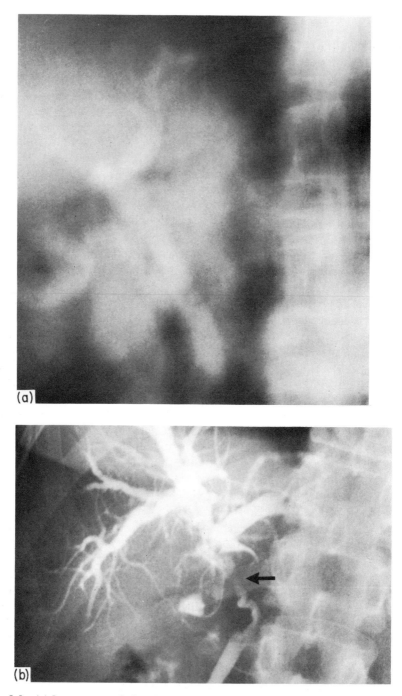

Fig. 5.5 *(a) Intravenous cholangiogram, note the poor definition of the common bile duct detail. (b) Percutaneous transhepatic cholangiogram, note good definition of the biliary system, dilated intrahepatic bile ducts and non-dilated common bile duct. Here is a block at porta hepatis (arrowed).*

some patients. Improvements in technique such as a prolonged infusion of the dye or tomograms of the common bile duct have marginally improved the use of the technique. Alternatively, abdominal ultrasonography used in conjunction with percutaneous transhepatic cholangiography (PTC) or endoscopic retrograde cholangiopancreatography (ERCP) have greatly improved identification of the common bile duct and its lesions and is gradually superseding intravenous cholangiography in the jaundiced and non-jaundiced patient (Fig. 5.5(a)).

PTC is of great value in detecting the site of obstruction in the jaundiced patient. The technique has become practicable and safe as a result of development of the Chiba needle in Japan. This 'skinny' needle means that the dilated intrahepatic bile ducts may be penetrated with safety until bile can be seen to be flowing back up the needle. Thereafter, the radiologist can inject radio-opaque dye which then fills the dilated biliary system above the level of obstruction. Excellent definition may thus be obtained with minimum discomfort to the patient. Where available, this technique has largely superseded intravenous cholangiography in the investigation of the jaundiced patient in whom ultrasonography has previously demonstrated the presence of a dilated biliary system. In the non-dilated biliary system the technique is more difficult since the radiologist has greater difficulty in penetrating an intrahepatic bile duct. Nevertheless, in skilled radiological hands, filling of the non-dilated biliary system can still be obtained. Techniques have recently been developed whereby palliative prostheses may be inserted across inoperable benign or malignant strictures of the biliary system via the percutaneous transhepatic route. In some patients with obstructive jaundice, both PTC and endoscopic retrograde cholangiography may be necessary to assess the full extent and nature of strictures in the common bile duct (Fig. 5.5(b)).

Endoscopic retrograde cholangiography is of great value in the investigation of suspected bile duct pathology. It may be combined with retrograde pancreatography. With increasing use of ultrasonography and PTC, retrograde cholangiography has an established role in the investigation of the non-jaundiced patient in whom biliary disease is suspected but unproven by other means. In the technique, the ampulla of Vater is identified endoscopically using a side-viewing duodenoscope. The papilla can then be cannulated with a 2 mm polythene cannula passed via the biopsy channel of the endoscope. Prior filling of the cannula with dye will usually ensure that no air bubbles are introduced into the biliary system to produce artefactual effects. It is often useful to use half-strength dye in the first instance since full concentration may obscure the presence of small bile duct stones. Good filling of the biliary system can be obtained by this means and the presence of a radiologist during the procedure aids interpretation of the abnormalities identified (Fig. 5.6).

Extension of the basic diagnostic technique of ERCP to encompass endoscopic papillotomy requires skill and experience and should only be undertaken once this level of expertise has been attained and the team is well versed in the

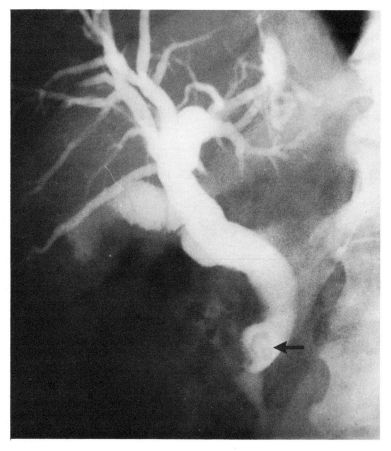

Fig. 5.6 *Endoscopic retrograde cholangiogram. Endoscope removed, note the stone in the distal common bile duct (arrowed) and dilated biliary system.*

procedure. Additional equipment, namely a diathermy source and papillotomy 'knives', will have to be provided. The basic technique is as for ERCP but selective cannulation of the common bile duct must be undertaken with the papillotomy 'knife' and will have to be confirmed radiologically before the papillotomy cut is undertaken. Endoscopic papillotomy is an ideal technique for the removal of common bile duct stones retained after cholecystectomy or even with the gall bladder still in place in the elderly patient with obstructive jaundice due to gall-stones in the common bile duct. After the papillotomy cut has been performed, extraction of the retained stones may be undertaken with a balloon catheter or a Dormia basket passed down the channel of the endoscope. A further refinement of the technique is to use an extremely long fine polythene cannula which may be inserted deep into the common bile duct and left there once the endoscope has been removed. Simple manipulations can bring this cannula out

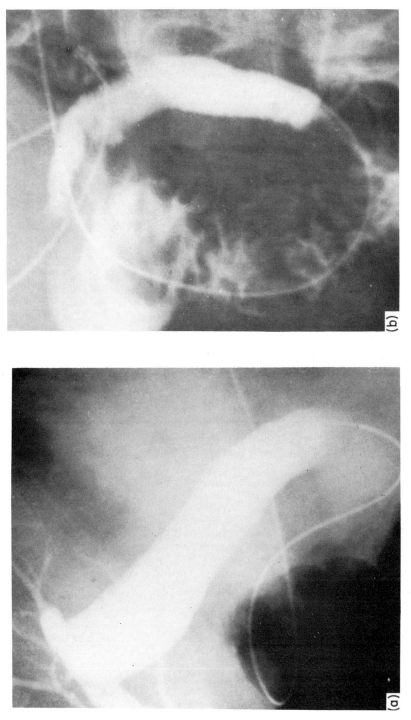

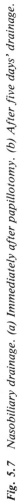

Fig. 5.7 Nasobiliary drainage. (a) Immediately after papillotomy. (b) After five days' drainage.

through the nose (so called nasobiliary cannulation). This technique means that repeat retrograde cholangiography may be performed without resort to endoscopy. It also means that the common bile duct may be irrigated with solutions to dissolve common bile duct stones in circumstances where their successful extraction post-papillotomy has not been achieved (Fig. 5.7). ERCP is also required if the insertion of a palliative prosthesis into the lower end of the common bile duct is contemplated. Future development of endoscopic retrograde techniques may see the availability of balloon catheters for dilatation of benign strictures of the common bile duct. To date, such procedures are still in the process of development and research evaluation.

The techniques described above apply to the patient in whom conventional anatomy is still present and where the route to the second part of the duodenum is through the pylorus. It is much more difficult to approach the ampulla in a retrograde manner up the afferent loop in patients who have undergone previous gastric surgery. This requires an even greater degree of skill and may sometimes best be achieved using an end-viewing rather than a side-viewing endoscope.

Transplenic portal venography is a technique in which a fine needle is introduced into the parenchyma of the spleen, through which radio-opaque dye can

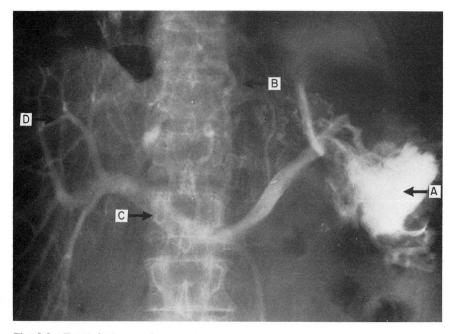

Fig. 5.8   *Transplenic portal venogram. A, Dye in splenic pulp; B, variceal collaterals; C, large portal vein; D, abnormal hepatic vasculature.*

be injected. This is a valuable technique for identifying patency of the splenic vein and portal venous system in patients with suspected portal hypertension and splenomegaly. It is an essential preliminary to the consideration of any portacaval anastomotic operation even though with the development of endoscopic sclerotherapy for patients with bleeding oesophageal varices, portacaval anastomotic procedures have reduced in numbers. The technique remains invaluable for imaging of the portal venous sytem and assessment of patency of the portal vein. (Fig. 5.8).

Angiography of the hepatic arterial system using a technique of selective cannulation of the coeliac axis may be useful in delineating the extent of hepatic tumours prior to consideration for surgery or chemotherapy.

Ultrasonography

There has been progressive improvement in the quality of imaging produced by ultrasonic scanners. As a result, where the technique is available, ultrasonography has become the primary non-invasive investigation of patients with jaundice. Ultrasonic scanning of the liver is able to identify whether or not intrahepatic bile ducts are dilated, the presence of intrahepatic tumours, and the presence of gallstones in both the gall bladder and the biliary system. A skilled ultrasonographer can also identify the presence of structural abnormalities in the pancreas. An additional benefit of the technique is the facility to insert a fine needle into a suspicious lesion under direct ultrasonic control. Aspiration of the contents of such lesions for cytology can be a valuable aid to diagnosis. The availability of ultrasonography has significantly altered the methods of investigation of the jaundiced patient (Fig. 5.9).

Isotopic liver scans

Radionuclide imaging is a simple technique used in the detection of focal hepatic disease. Lesions usually have to exceed 2–4 cm in diameter to be seen although patchy uptake by the spleen and bone marrow are characteristic of cirrhosis with portal hypertension. The most commonly used isotope is technetium sulphur colloid (^{99m}Tc) which is taken up by the reticuloendothelial cells. Scanning can thereafter be performed with a mobile counting head or static pictures may be taken with a gamma camera. Alternatively, HIDA (^{99m}Tc) or technetium tin collid (^{99m}Tc) may be used. Apart from the intravenous injection of the isotope, the techniques are non-invasive and the patient need not be starved for prolonged periods of time. The procedure usually takes no longer than an hour.

Some radioisotopes are excreted by liver cells after intravenous injection. The use of technetium ^{99m}HIDA or DISIDA (iminodiacetate complexes) forms the basis of an isotope test in the jaundiced patient. Non-visualization of the gall bladder by isotope scanning within four hours of intravenous injection of ^{99m}Tc HIDA is suggestive of gall bladder disease as the cause of jaundice.

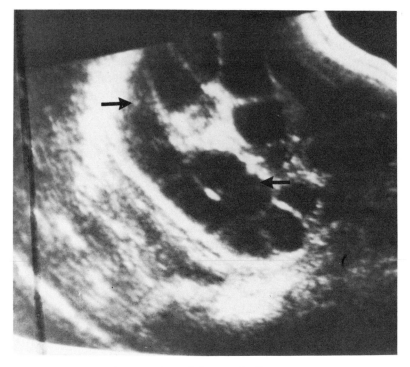

Fig. 5.9   Ultrasonography, note large defects in the liver.

Whole body scanning or computerized tomography is a specialized radiological technique which produces very clear pictures of the texture of the liver and its surrounding organs. Isotopes may be used in whole body scanning to give clearer definition. Computerized tomography is an advanced technique which requires very expensive equipment which is not always available.

Liver biopsy

This is a simple and safe procedure when performed by an experienced clinician. Various types of needle are now available, the best being the disposable pre-sterilized type. The commonest technique is to insert the needle into the liver through an intercostal space in the lateral chest wall under local anaesthetic. An alternative approach is the subcostal route through the anterior abdominal wall in the right upper quadrant of the abdomen over the surface of the enlarged liver. Both techniques require a co-operative patient who is able to stop breathing whilst the biopsy is taken. Coagulation factors must be checked prior to the procedure. Afterwards, the patient remains in bed for 24 hours and a regular check is maintained upon pulse and blood pressure measurements. As an additional precaution in case of a post-procedure haemorrhage, the blood group of the patient should be known and blood for transfusion should be readily available. Mild abdominal or shoulder-tip pain is common after the procedure, whilst bleeding or biliary leakage leading to peritonitis are rare complications (Fig. 5.10).

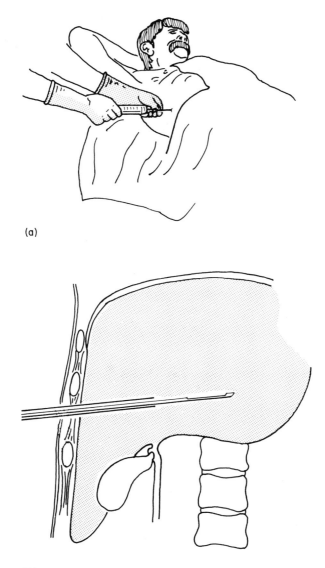

(a)

(b)

Fig. 5.10 *Liver biopsy technique. (a) The patient lies comfortably with his right side on the edge of the bed. (b) The biopsy needle passes into the liver substance through an intercostal space.*

Liver biopsy yields only a small sample of liver so that only in patients with diffuse liver disease are the most representative results obtained. Biopsy is essential in the diagnosis of chronic hepatitis and in establishing a diagnosis of cirrhosis. Features indicating alcohol abuse or haemochromatosis may also be identified histologically. Liver biopsy is not usually required in acute hepatitis in which the diagnosis can normally be made on other grounds, although in atypical cases histological features may be beneficial. Liver biopsy is of little value in elucidating causes of obstructive jaundice where other techniques are more satisfactory. Localized disease, especially malignancy, is best diagnosed by liver biopsy or aspiration under controlled conditions using ultrasonography to guide the biopsy needle into position. Pre-operative liver biopsy may sometimes be of value in the staging of lymphoma.

Laparoscopy

Laparoscopy is a technique in which the intra-abdominal cavity can be inspected via a laparoscope introduced through the anterior abdominal wall under local or general anaesthesia. Nitrous oxide or carbon dioxide is insufflated into the abdominal cavity to separate the anterior abdominal wall from the organs. Laparoscopy provides an excellent view of the anterior and superior surfaces of the liver and the gall bladder whilst the spleen and omental surfaces can be readily seen. Biopsy forceps pass down the laparoscope and can provide tissue for diagnosis from involved areas in suspected malignant disease. Laparoscopy is contraindicated when there are haemostatic abnormalities, gross ascites and previous surgery which may have caused abdominal adhesions. The laparoscope is of little value in identifying pancreatic or small intestinal pathology.

Investigation of the jaundiced patient

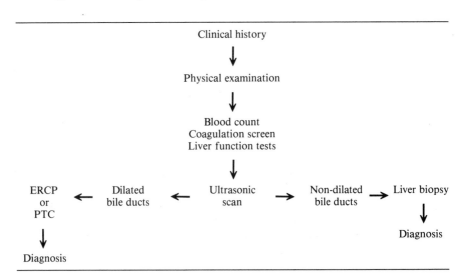

NURSING CARE DURING INVESTIGATION AND THERAPEUTIC PROCEDURES

Endoscopic retrograde cholangiography

At least two nurses are required to ensure that this procedure is carried out safely and satisfactorily. Hospital admission for the patient should be arranged if requested by the clinician.

Check list

As for routine gastrointestinal endoscopy plus:
A side-viewing endoscope with forceps raiser. Check the forceps raiser is functioning correctly before use and lubricate control and distal tip with silicone fluid to ensure that it will continue to operate satisfactorily.

Endoscopic cannulae for injection of contrast medium. These cannulae should be clean, disinfected or sterilized, dry and patent before use. A guide-wire may be integral or separate and must be smooth to allow free passage of the cannula down the biopsy channel (Fig. 5.11).

Radiographic contrast medium of choice

20 or 30 ml syringes

Filling tubes for drawing up

Sodium chloride 0.9% to dilute the contrast

Antifoam agent to reduce bile bubbles and improve the endoscopist's view. This may be administered orally prior to the procedure (10 ml should be sufficient) or it may be injected via a cannula through the endoscope (Table 5.1)

Intravenous cannulae for the administration of drugs

Intravenous drugs: see Table 5.2

Further requirements:
Check availability of radiology screening facilities

Check the 10-day rule if appropriate

If image intensification facilities are not available in the Gastroenterology department, arrange safe transfer of all equipment required to the Radiology department

Procedure

On receiving the patient, the nurse must ensure that the procedure is understood and that informed written consent has been obtained by the referring clinician. Premedication is given if prescribed. Local anaesthesia to the throat is administered as for routine oesophagogastroduodenoscopy.

The patient is positioned on the radiography table on the left side with the left arm behind the back, before sedation is administered. This makes it easier to

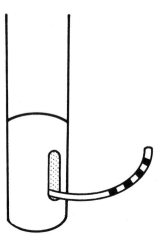

Fig. 5.11   *ERCP cannula protruding through the biopsy channel port of a side-viewing duodenoscope.*

turn the patient prone during the procedure as this may be required to facilitate cannulation of the duct system (Fig. 5.12).

An intravenous cannula is inserted into the back of the right hand. Some endoscopists prefer to establish an intravenous infusion prior to the procedure. This may then be used for the administration of sedation, resuscitation in the event of complications and antibiotics in a septic case. The i.v. line may be discontinued immediately after the procedure if not required.

Table 5.1

De-foaming agent
Silicone fluid MS 200/500 − 10 ml
Fused silica powder 0.5 g
Mannitol 140 g
Dose 5 ml to 1 l H_2O
Method: 1 level teaspoon injected down channel or taken orally

DC Antifoam Emulsion M30
Formula:

| DC Antifoam Emulsion M30* | | 1.5 g | i.e. 0.15% |
| Purified water | to | 1 l | |

Method: Take the balance with a 1 l measure and weigh 1.5 g of DC Antifoam Emulsion into this. Add about 800 ml purified water to the measure and stir quickly. Make up to volume with purified water. When made up to volume, mix using Silverson mixer with fine mesh attachment for a couple of minutes
Container: 1 l amber medicine bottle, screw cap and white visk ring. Better in 20−25 ml bottles
Expiry: 4 weeks

---

* Supplied by Hopkin & Williams, Chadwell Heath, Essex, England.

Commercially available de-foaming agents may also be used, and they require no pre-mixing.

Table 5.2   Drugs which may be required during ERCP

I.V. Diazepam
I.V. Pethidine
I.V. Naloxone (Narcan)
I.V. Fortral
I.V. Hyoscine butyl bromide (Buscopan)
I.V. Glucagon
I.V. Secretin
I.V. Pancreozymin
Water for injection
I.V. antibiotics should be readily available as they may be required in a septic case or
   should the patient's condition indicate

It may be necessary to give extra sedation in order to keep the patient more
comfortable during this longer and more complicated procedure. A usual combination may be:

   I.V. Diazepam in titrated doses
      plus either
   I.V. Pethidine in titrated doses
      or
   I.V. Fortral in titrated doses

Intravenous Hyoscine butyl bromide (Buscopan) may be given now or when
the endoscopist requests it, most likely when the endoscope is in the duodenum.
If there is excess foaming of bile bubbles in the duodenum antifoam agent can
now be injected down a cannula or the wash tube attachment.

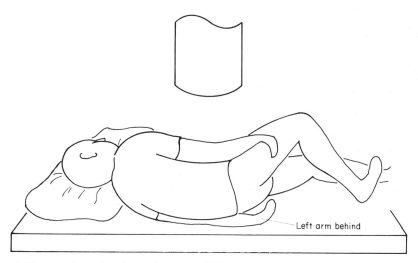

Left arm behind

Fig. 5.12   *Position of patient prior to ERCP/sphincterotomy. Note left arm behind to
facilitate easy change of position from left lateral to prone.*

The cannulae to be used should be pre-filled, with care being taken to expel all air bubbles as these give misleading information during radiological screening. At least two syringes of contrast should be available to prevent delay when more is required. It may be necessary to use large quantities of contrast in a dilated system and after sphincterotomy. In order to visualize small stones in ducts, dilute contrast may be required, e.g. 50% contrast and 50% sterile sodium chloride 0.9%, as full strength contrast may be too dense.

When requested the cannula is passed to the endoscopist who will introduce it via the biopsy channel of the duodenoscope into the papilla. This is done with the syringe attached to the cannula. When the syringe is changed over for a fresh one, it is advisable to pull back slightly on the piston to ensure that no air passes into the ducts. Injection of the contrast is done by the assisting nurse. Syringe sizes of 20–30 ml are easier to use than larger syringes.

The patient is reassured during the procedure and kept in the correct position. Radiological screening is used and radiographs are taken during the procedure. Alterations to the position of the patient may be required in order to obtain better views. It is also usual to take radiographs after removal of the endoscope as this may be overlying part of the duct system.

After the procedure, the patient is made comfortable in bed. Any special instructions should be carried out.

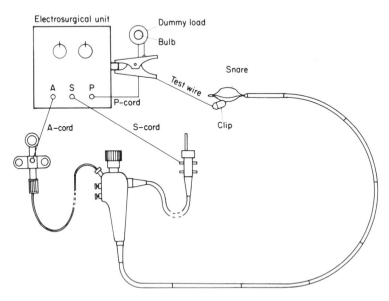

Fig. 5.13 *Checking the diathermy unit using a dummy load. A-cord: to accessory; S-cord: to 'scope; P-cord: to patient (NB: S- and P-cords may be a joint cord going to one socket).*

Endoscopic sphincterotomy (papillotomy)

This procedure is exactly as for endoscopic cholangiography with the addition of diathermy to the ampulla of Vater.

Check list

Diathermy unit: check before use (Fig. 5.13)
Sphincterotomes: one per patient plus spare wires (Fig. 5.14)
Stone retrieval baskets (Fig. 5.15)
Balloon catheters (Fig. 5.16)
Polythene drainage tubing: one length per patient, at least twice the length of the endoscope

Procedure

After visualization of stones in the common bile duct on radiological screening at endoscopic cholangiography, the sphincterotome is passed via the endoscope biopsy channel and introduced into the ampulla of Vater. The assisting nurse is

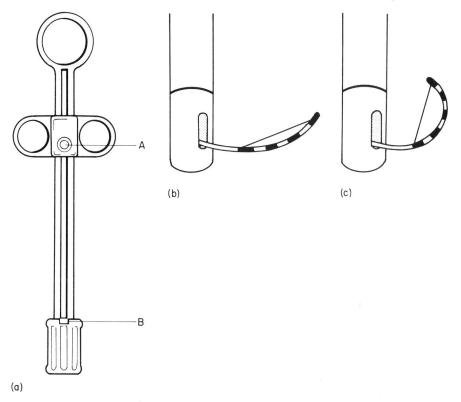

Fig. 5.14 *(a) Diathermy handle showing (A) connection to A-cord and (B) locking system. (b) Papillotome straight and (c) bowed.*

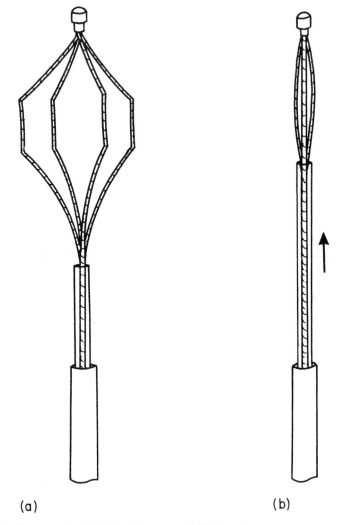

(a)   (b)

Fig. 5.15   *Stone retrieval basket (a) open and (b) closed.*

responsible for adjusting the wire as requested by the endoscopist. If it is necessary to keep the stones adequately visualized contrast may be introduced via the sphincterotome. The nurse will also be required to control the supply of current from the diathermy unit and should ensure that the correct amount is used by ascertaining through verbal repetition that she has understood the endoscopist's instructions.

The patient must be reassured during this process as it is possible for some transient discomfort to be felt. After successful sphincterotomy, the endoscopist may either remove stones with the aid of a basket or a balloon catheter,

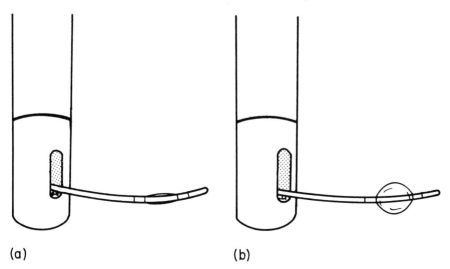

(a)   (b)

Fig. 5.16 *Endoscopic balloon catheter (a) deflated and (b) inflated.*

or insert a biliary drainage tube into the duct via the biopsy channel and remove the endoscope over the tube. As this tube may be left in place for some time, it should be rerouted via the nose − see 'Nasobiliary drainage' p. 158−60.

Visualization of the duct to ascertain the success of the procedure may take place immediately by further injection of contrast via the drainage tube or the balloon catheter, which has a double lumen, or by using a fresh cannula via the endoscope then or at a later date.

After removal of the endoscope the patient is made comfortable. Any antibiotic therapy is given and recovery should take place under careful observation as for post-endoscopic cholangiography, with particular attention paid for signs of post-procedure haemorrhage and infection.

Complication of ERCP and sphincterotomy

Simple visualization of the ducts is a safe procedure and complications are rare. Occasionally cholangitis and septicaemia may follow manipulation in an obstructed common bile duct, whilst over-filling of the pancreatic duct or a pancreatic pseudo-cyst during the procedure may precipitate an attack of pancreatitis.

With encoscopic sphincterotomy bleeding, perforation and impaction of stone or basket may occur as immediate complications of the procedure. Fortunately, torrential bleeding at the time is a rare complication, and is usually precipitated by cutting into an aberrant artery. Late bleeding, after 3−4 days, is an even more rare complication. Surgery will be necessary for all significant bleeding since endoscopic techniques are inadequate to arrest the haemorrhage. Once again pancreatitis may occur.

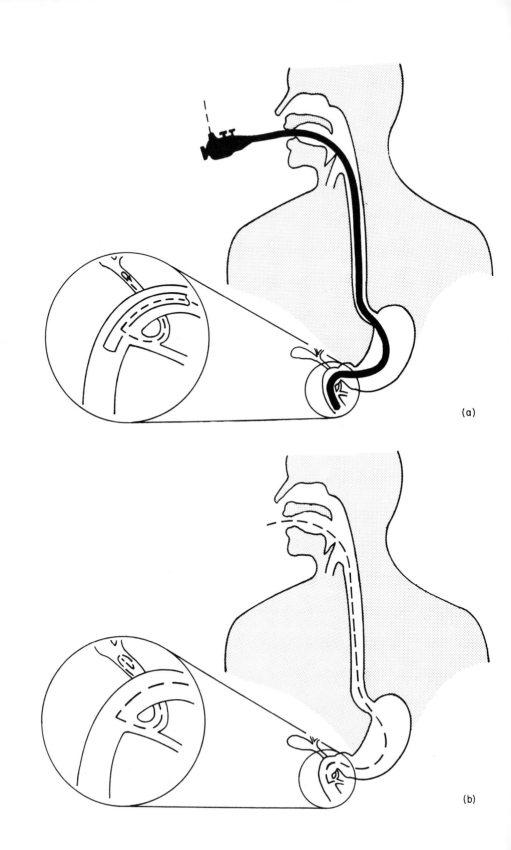

(a)

(b)

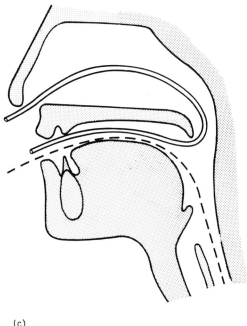

(c)

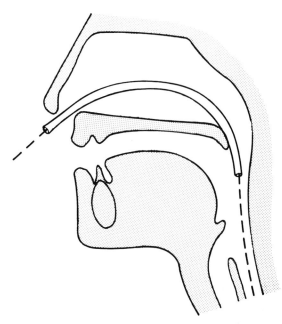

(d)

Fig. 5.17 *The technique of nasobiliary drainage. (a) A 3 m length of fine polythene tubing is passed into the common bile duct via the endoscope. (b) Under radiological control, the endoscope is removed, taking care to leave the fine tube in position. (c) A nasogastric tube is passed via the nose and brought out through the mouth. (d) The fine polytheme tube is threaded retrograde up the nasogastric tube which can then be removed. Nasobiliary intubation is achieved.*

Instructions for the introduction and care of a nasobiliary drainage tube

Check list

Sterilized polythene drainage tubing 6F gauge outer diameter
14F gauge nasogastric tube
Torch
Spatulae
Laryngoscope
Forceps
Scissors
Adhesive tape
Black silk
Luer end
Drainage bag
Lubricant
Gauze swabs

Procedure

Before use, the tubing may have lateral drainage holes cut into the distal end to allow for free drainage of secretions from the bile duct. When in place it can either be fastened off and used only for injection of contrast or it can be attached to a collecting bag to allow for free drainage of bile.

The tube will initially come out through the patient's mouth, on removal of the endoscope. As it may be left in place for some time, it requires to be re-routed through the nose in order that the patient may eat and drink normally. This is done by passing a lubricated 14F gauge nasogastric tube into the hypopharynx and with the aid of a torch and spatula or a laryngoscope, the distal tip of the nasogastric tube is located and withdrawn through the mouth with a pair of forceps. The tip is then cut off and the drainage tube threaded out through the nasogastric tube. It is pulled gently until it is comfortably situated at the back of the throat, the nasogastric tube is withdrawn and the drainage tube cut to the required length. The patient is given advice on what to expect with this tube in place. There may be some minor throat discomfort and green or yellow fluid may appear in the tube. Also, some movement of the tube may be experienced when eating and drinking (Fig. 5.17).

The patient is reassured and given a further appointment for repeat nasobiliary cholangiography and any subsequent investigation or treatment.

Insertion of endoscopic biliary prosthesis

This procedure may include endoscopic cholangiography, pancreatography, and sphincterotomy.

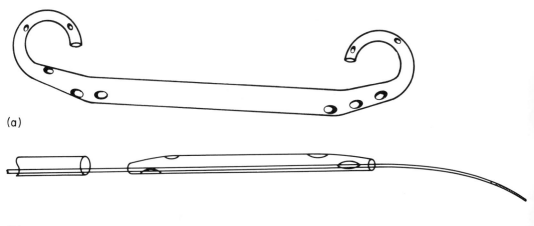

(a)

(b)

Fig. 5.18 *(a) 'Pig tail' biliary prosthesis. (b) Guide-wire, prosthesis and pusher.*

Check list

Equipment is required as for ERCP and sphincterotomy plus:
Biliary prosthesis with introducers – more than one may be introduced depending on the clinician's requirements. The size will also be a matter of choice e.g. 6, 8 or 10F. This also depends on the diameter of the biopsy channel of the endoscope. Biopsy forceps may be required to remove previous or unsatisfactorily placed prostheses (Fig. 5.18)

Procedure

After satisfactory sphincterotomy, the prosthesis and introducer are threaded down the biopsy channel of the endoscope. The prosthesis is positioned in the common bile duct under radiological control, care being taken to ensure that it straddles the obstructive lesion and a flow of bile is seen endoscopically. A second prosthesis may be introduced in the same way.

Antibiotic therapy is likely to be initiated if it has not already been prescribed. Patients undergoing this procedure are likely to be terminally ill and require skilled nursing care. Repeat abdominal radiology and duodenoscopy will be required to monitor the efficacy of this procedure. In the event of recurrence of jaundice, blockage of the prosthesis may have occurred, thus requiring a repeat of the procedure to insert a fresh prosthesis (Fig. 5.19).

Liver biopsy

This is an aseptic procedure carried out by a doctor with a nurse to assist. The patient is usually admitted on the day before the procedure is to take place when

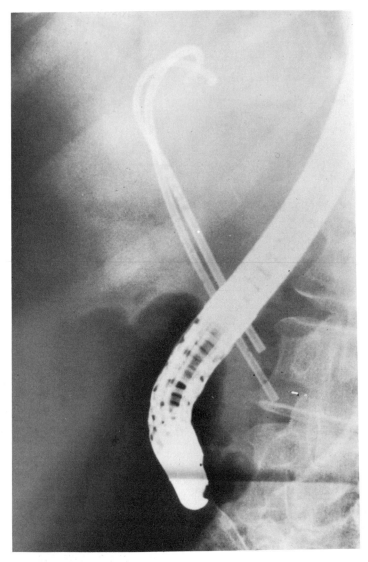

Fig. 5.19   *Biliary prostheses in place.*

the following blood tests should be done and their results checked before the biopsy is performed:

Prothrombin index (PI)
Partial thromboplastin time (PTT)
Platelet count
Blood group, crossmatch and hold serum

(Some of these tests may have been done before the patient is admitted to hospital.)

Check list

A trolley is cleaned and prepared for aseptic technique
5 ml syringe
Hypodermic needles, large and small size
Local anaesthetic
Cotton wool balls or gauze squares
Absorbent sterile towels
Sterile gloves − size of choice
Skin preparation
Scalpel blade
Needle for biopsy (Menghini, Tru-cut or Gilman)
Paper for mounting liver sample
Specimen container with 10% formalin − labelled correctly
Histology form
Small adhesive plaster dressings

Procedure

The procedure is explained to the patient, reassurance given and co-operation gained. Informed written consent should be obtained by the referring clinician and checked by the nurse. Blood pressure and pulse rate are taken and recorded. The trolley is taken to the right side of the bed which should be screened from the main ward area. While the doctor washes his hands, the assistant positions the patient.

The patient lies flat along the right edge of the bed with one pillow supporting the head and the right arm behind the head. This makes the liver more accessible for the biopsy.

The assistant wipes the trolley top with the alcohol wipe, opens the dressing packs onto it and discards the wrappers. The doctor dries his hands with a sterile towel, puts on the gloves and arranges the equipment. The assistant pours skin preparation into the container provided. The doctor arranges the sterile towels, identifies the biopsy site and marks it. The local anaesthetic is then drawn up into the 5 ml syringe and the area over the biopsy site anaesthetized.

With a scalpel blade the doctor makes a small incision at the chosen site and asks the patient to stop breathing whilst the biopsy needle is inserted. The liver specimen is aspirated and placed on the mounting paper which is then put into the formalin-filled specimen container.

The doctor places a swab over the puncture wound until local bleeding ceases and then cleans and dries the area before applying a small adhesive dressing to the wound. The patient is repositioned in the centre of the bed and made comfortable.

Disposable equipment is discarded. The labelled specimen with completed request card are sent to the Histopathology laboratory.

After the procedure, the patient remains on bed rest for 24 hours. Blood pressure and pulse recordings are taken every 30 minutes for the next two hours and every 60 minutes for the following six hours. The puncture site is checked at these intervals for signs of bleeding. These recorded observations are necessary in case internal bleeding should occur.

Complications of liver biopsy

Patients frequently complain of abdominal or shoulder-tip pain. This is due to diaphragmatic irritation and is usually controlled by simple analgesics. The development of hypotension and more severe pain suggest the rare complications of haemorrhage or biliary peritonitis post-biopsy. The doctor should be kept informed of such developments, which usually settle with conservative management.

LAPAROSCOPY

Laparoscopy is a technique for inspection of the organs within the abdominal cavity. Using a rigid fibreoptic laparoscope introduced through the anterior abdominal wall, the clinician can inspect the organs of the pelvis, the mesentery, the gall bladder, liver surface and pancreas. Biopsies of suspicious lesions and operative techniques may be undertaken through the instrument. The technique is useful to gastroenterologists and gynaecologists, for whom it is of particular value in the investigation of abnormal masses, suspected intra-abdominal malignancy and pancreatic disease. It is usually performed as an inpatient procedure and coagulation studies and cross matching will usually have been performed beforehand.

Procedure

The procedure should be explained to the patient and written informed consent obtained by the medical staff and checked by nursing staff. Premedication with diazepam or pethidine will usually have been given one hour before the procedure.

With the patient comfortably positioned in the prone position an indwelling intravenous needle is inserted and secured. Intravenous diazepam (10–20 mg) is given by slow intravenous injection until the patient is adequately sedated.

The abdomen is exposed and cleansed with a skin preparation fluid. Sterile drapes are positioned with a towel rail in place to keep the sterile drapes off the face of the patient. Two sites on the anterior abdominal wall are then anaesthetized using 2% lignocaine. The first site is in the area of the left iliac fossa; the second site subumbilically in the mid-line.

With the anterior abdominal wall suitably anaesthetized a Verres needle is inserted through a small incision made in the anterior abdominal wall. A 20 ml syringe is attached to this needle and aspiration performed to exclude intestinal or large vessel perforation. Once this has been performed a generous pneumo-peritoneum should be induced using nitrous oxide. When the abdomen is dis-tended and tympanitic, the second incision is made below the umbilicus.

At this point, the patient is asked to tense the abdominal wall and the laparo-scopic trocar and cannula are inserted through this incision. The trocar is removed and the pre-heated laparoscope inserted through the cannula. Once the light guide has been attached, the site of insertion of the Verres needle should be inspected internally to exclude significant internal haemorrhage at this site. The Verres needle should now be withdrawn and the insufflation tubing transferred to the laparoscopic cannula. A full examination of the liver, gall bladder, pancreas, omentum and pelvis may now be made.

If biopsies are required from the liver or suspicious lesions, a specially designed long biopsy needle may be passed down the channel of the laparo-scope. Aspiration or punch biopsies of the lesion may be obtained. Once this is performed, the specimen is expelled from the needle onto a specimen card for transfer to the Histopathology department. The site of internal biopsy may be inspected for evidence of secondary haemorrhage.

Once the examination is completed, the laparoscope is withdrawn and the pneumoperitoneum reduced. The subumbilical incision is closed in two layers and both insertion sites cleaned and simple dressings applied. Should ascites be present, additional pressure dressings will be required.

The patient should be reassured, made comfortable and returned to a recovery area with full nursing instructions.

Complications of laparoscopy

Abdominal discomfort is common after the procedure and is usually due to residual gaseous distension. Manipulation of adhesions during the procedure can also be painful. More persistent pain and peritonism suggest bleeding from a biopsy site or the development of a haematoma within peritoneal ligaments or mesentery. Hypotension and shock suggest that more copious haemorrhage has occurred. The doctor must be informed.

Check list

Drugs: diazepam
       naloxone (Narcan)
Intravenous cannulae
Tourniquet
Alcohol wipes
Gauze swabs
Light source

continued

Insufflator with nitrous oxide gas cylinder attached
Carbon dioxide cylinder with flow meter and gauge
Bowl of sterile water
Pre-heater
Procedure trolley — top shelf is a sterile area. On this lay up:
   One laparoscopy pack — opened using aseptic technique
   Add: Scalpel blade (23)
        Suture materials — Chromic and Mersilk 2/0
        10 ml syringes
        20 ml syringe
        Needles
        Trocar and cannula
        Light carrier
        Teaching attachment
        Laparoscope
        Menghini needle
        Tactile probe
        Verres needle
        Insufflation tubing
        Insertion tubes for pre-heater
   Bottom shelf is unsterile:
        Skin cleansing solutions
        Lignocaine 2%
        Sodium chloride 0.9%
        Specimen container
        Specimen card or ground glass cover slip
        Plastic skin dressing
        Elastoplast dressings
        Spare syringes and needles
        Histology request form

Ideally, one hour before the procedure, the sterile insertion tube should be placed in the pre-heater and the sterile laparoscope should be rinsed thoroughly in sterile water and dried with sterile absorbent towels. When dry, it should be placed in the pre-heater and covered with sterile towels

Additional requirements:
   Resuscitation equipment
   Suction apparatus
   Oxygen

Contents of laparoscopy pack:
   1 receiver containing 2 gallipots and 1 sponge-holder
   Scalpel handle
   8 towel clips
   2 mosquito artery forceps
   1 plain dissecting forceps

continued

1 rat-toothed dissecting forceps
1 stitch holder
4 drapes
Gauze swabs × 10
1 gallipot
1 pair of scissors

6

THE PANCREAS

ANATOMY

The pancreas is an important accessory gland to the digestive system. Its structure is somewhat similar to that of the salivary glands. It lies across the posterior abdominal wall at the level of the first and second lumbar vertebrae and is situated behind the stomach. It has a head, a body and a tail. The head is situated to the right of the vertebral column and sits snuggly into the curvature of the duodenum. Buried deep in the substance of the gland in this area is the common bile duct which joins the pancreatic duct to form the ampulla of Vater which opens into the medial wall of the duodenum and is protected by a muscular band, the sphincter of Oddi. The body of the pancreas is about 30 cm long and runs transversely across the vertebral column towards the left. The terminal part of the body is called the tail and is in close contact with the hilum of the spleen. Posteriorly, the pancreas sits on the great vessels, the lumbar vertebrae and the posterior abdominal wall. The anterior surface of the gland is covered by peritoneum and is overlaid by the body of the stomach. The splenic artery and vein run along its upper surface (Fig. 6.1).

The gland is constructed of a number of lobules formed by secretory tubules lined with columnar epithelium. The small ductules draining each lobule gradually unite and eventually reach the main pancreatic duct which runs through the centre of the organ. This passes throughout the body of the pancreas and joins the common bile duct in the head before entering the medial wall of the second part of the duodenum in the ampulla of Vater. Between the clumps of secretory tubules or acini, are collections of cells of differing structure called the islets of Langerhans which mainly secrete insulin.

PHYSIOLOGY

The pancreas has two different types of secretion. The exocrine or external secretion is produced in the secretory tubules and leaves the gland via the

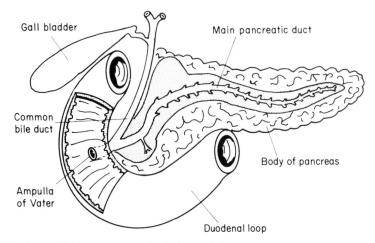

Fig. 6.1   *Anatomical structure and relations of the pancreas.*

pancreatic duct. This external secretion is an important digestive juice and contains several constituents:

Amylase − which converts starches to maltose
Lipase − which splits fat into fatty acids and glycerol
Trypsin − which converts peptides into amino acids
Bicarbonate − which neutralizes gastric acid in the upper gastrointestinal tract

All of these constituents are secreted in a fluid volume of approximately a litre daily. The enzymes enter the duodenum via the pancreatic duct and mix with food which has left the stomach. They continue to act on gastrointestinal contents during passage through the small intestine. The pancreas also produces insulin from the islets of Langerhans. This is absorbed directly into the bloodstream and is the endocrine production of the pancreas.

Acid, fat and hypertonic solutions in the duodenum release the hormones secretin and cholecystokinin from the duodenal mucosa into the bloodstream. Secretin stimulates the secretary acinar cells of the pancreas to produce bicarbonate and fluid. The enzymes amylase, lipase and trypsin are produced in response to cholecystokinin−pancreozymin release.

PATHOLOGY (Fig. 6.2)

Acute pancreatitis

This is a serious disorder caused by autodigestion of the pancreas by its own enzymes. It usually presents as an acute abdominal catastrophe and whereas in

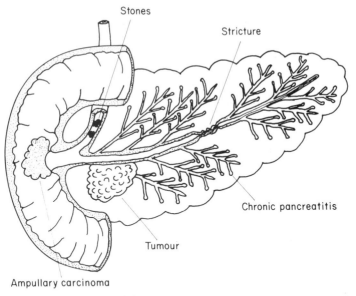

Stones

Stricture

Chronic pancreatitis

Tumour

Ampullary carcinoma

Fig. 6.2   Important disorders of the pancreas.

mild cases the gland becomes swollen and oedematous, in more severe cases, haemorrhagic necrosis occurs with the development of serious complications. Most commonly, the attack may be precipitated by biliary disease or alcohol. In about 20% of cases no cause can be identified. Acute pancreatitis is also a recognized complication of renal transplantation, steroid therapy, oral contraceptives and immunosuppressants. It may occasionally be produced by abdominal trauma, surgery, mumps, hyperparathyroidism, hyperlipidaemia or hypothermia.

The acute attack may be catastrophic and may present as an acute abdominal emergency. Indeed, the severity of the shock of the acute episode may be fatal. In milder cases, abdominal pain, fever and slight jaundice may develop. The importance of the milder attacks of acute pancreatitis is that they may go on to produce chronic pancreatitis with progressive destruction of the gland and subsequent calcification.

Investigation of the acute attack lies in measurement of serum and urinary amylase, plain radiography of the abdomen and ultrasonography of the pancreas. Monitoring of progress should include repeated estimation of serum amylase, serum electrolytes and blood glucose.

Chronic pancreatitis

In the Western world, the majority of cases of chronic pancreatitis occur as the result of high alcohol consumption. Rarely, the chronic state may be caused by recurrent acute pancreatitis, co-incidental gallstones or stenosis of the sphincter of Oddi. In underdeveloped countries, chronic pancreatitis is common and malnutrition is probably an important aetiological factor. In the chronic state, the body of the gland shows microscopical evidence of fibrosis around the ducts and acini which are gradually replaced by fibrous tissue and calcification. The larger ducts are often irregular and dilated and calculi may be present in the lumen. The pancreatic exocrine secretion gradually diminishes. By contrast, there is preservation of the islets of Langerhans and insulin production is maintained. The disease is most common in males between the age of 35 and 45 years. The most common presentation is with abdominal pain located in the epigastrium, sub-costal areas or around the umbilicus. Thirty per cent of patients develop steatorrhoea whilst 20% eventually develop diabetes. Jaundice may occur because of obstruction to the common bile duct with progressive fibrosis in the head of the pancreas which may become calcified.

In a small proportion of cases of chronic pancreatitis, the condition can be confirmed from plain radiography of the abdomen which shows calcification in the duct system or throughout the gland. Ultrasound of the pancreas is an invaluable investigation for detecting abnormalities in the gland. Evidence of pancreatic insufficiency is provided when pancreatic function tests reveal reduced concentration of amylase and bicarbonate in the secretions which gradually diminish in volume with advancing disease. The presence of steatorrhoea and a diabetic glucose tolerance test provide further evidence of pancreatic insufficiency. Occasionally, endoscopic retrograde pancreatography may show minor disorganization of the glandular system which has not been detected by other means and may also show stones and dilatation of the duct system. The endoscopic retrograde technique may also be valuable for the performance of a papillotomy.

Carcinoma of the pancreas

The incidence of carcinoma of the pancreas is increasing in Western countries. It is more common in males than in females and most commonly occurs between the ages of 55 and 70 years. Most of the cancers of the pancreas are adenocarcinomas arising from the duct system of the gland. Apart from carcinoma of the ampulla of Vater which may bleed or cause obstructive jaundice at an early stage, all cancers of the pancreas are advanced by the time they cause symptoms. Symptoms are characteristically very variable and of a non-specific nature. Epigastric pain of a dull boring quality radiating through to the back is the common presentation. The pain may be intensified by food, worse at night and relieved by crouching forward. In the majority of cases, with involvement of the head of the pancreas, jaundice is the presenting feature and is usually painless and progressive. By the time jaundice presents, the primary growth has already metastasized and a large liver is commonly present. Sometimes, a palpable gall bladder or ascites can be detected. Occasionally, the symptoms of diabetes mellitus or thrombophlebitis may be the presenting feature. Because of the late manifestation of symptoms of the disease, curative surgery is not possible although a bypass operation may be performed to minimize the obstructive jaundice. The condition is rapidly progressive and death usually occurs within 6 months of the onset of obstructive jaundice.

Pancreatic cysts

Pancreatic pseudocysts occur as a complication of acute pancreatitis, chronic pancreatitis or injury to the pancreas. A pancreatic pseudocyst is a sac which contains fluid, pancreatic enzymes and blood. It may be large enough to displace the stomach and cause obstruction to the duodenum. The most common presentation is with epigastric pain, nausea and vomiting, weight loss, jaundice and fever. With larger cysts, a smooth tender mass may be palpated in the upper abdomen. Ultrasound of the pancreas is the diagnostic method of choice and once detected, pseudocysts which fail to remit spontaneously are treated surgically by drainage into the stomach or small intestine. Smaller retention cysts may be found in chronic pancreatitis. They are usually multiple, and cause abdominal pain as part of the symptom complex of chronic pancreatitis. Because of their size, it is difficult to establish the diagnosis by ultrasonography and retrograde pancreatography may be necessary.

Cystic fibrosis

This autosomal recessive disease is the commonest serious genetic condition in the Western world. It is caused by generalized dysfunction of all exocrine glands especially those which secrete mucus. In the pancreas, blockage of the duct systems by viscid secretion causes cystic changes and progressive decline in function. Whilst the most common presentation in infancy is with repeated attacks of respiratory infection, defective pancreatic enzymes give rise to malabsorption of fat and progressive malnutrition. Complications include intussusception and obstruction due to faecal masses. In the child, the diagnosis is established by finding an increase in the concentration of sodium in the sweat to above 60 mmol per litre. After adolescence, the sweat test is difficult to interpret and the diagnosis is usually established on the clinical spectrum of chronic pulmonary disease, pancreatic insufficiency and a family history of cystic fibrosis.

Pancreatic tumours

A benign adenoma may arise from the beta cells of the islets of Langerhans and produce hyperinsulinism with attacks of spontaneous hypoglycaemia. These tumours are rare but even more rare are those tumours, usually of slow advancing malignancy, which occur from other islet cells and produce polypeptides such as gastrin or allied substances. In the Zollinger–Ellison syndrome, excessive gastrin is produced by the tumour which stimulates the parietal cells of the stomach. As a result, the patient suffers multiple peptic ulceration which may occur in unusual sites such as the jejunum or oesophagus. Often the patient has had previous surgery for peptic ulceration. Diarrhoea and steatorrhoea may accompany the peptic ulceration since pancreatic lipase is inactivated and bile acids are precipitated by an acid upper small intestinal intraluminal pH. The diagnosis should be suspected in all patients with unusual or severe peptic ulceration especially if coarse gastric mucosal folds are identified. Confirmation of the condition is by gastric acid analysis with a pentagastrin test where the secretory rate which is already high at basal level is not increased by pentagastrin injection. Serum gastrin levels can be measured by radioimmunoassay and will be found to be elevated.

INVESTIGATIONS OF SUSPECTED PANCREATIC DISEASE

Laboratory based tests:
  Serum amylase
  Urine amylase
  Ascitic amylase
  Sweat electrolyte test
Radiology based:
  Plain abdominal radiology
  Pancreatic ultrasonography
  Endoscopic retrograde pancreatography
  Pancreatic angiography
  Computerized tomography
Gastroenterology department based:
  Sweat electrolyte test
  Pancreatic function tests:
    'Tube' tests: Lundh meal
                  Secretin-stimulation test
                  ^{75}Se selenomethionine test
    Tubeless tests: PABA test
                    Cobalt isotope test
                    Fluorescein dilaurate test
  Endoscopic retrograde pancreatography

Laboratory based investigations

In attacks of pancreatitis, the pancreas leaks amylase into the general circulation. It may be measured in serum, urine or ascitic fluid. In severe attacks, serum amylase may become grossly elevated.

Radiological investigations

A plain abdominal radiograph may give indications of pancreatic calcification. Pancreatic ultrasonography will show the shape and size of the pancreas and identify the presence of tumours, cysts or dilated ducts. It is a particularly useful test when carcinoma of the pancreas is suspected and has become the primary investigation of structural abnormalities of the pancreas.

Alternatively, endoscopic retrograde pancreatography may be undertaken. In this technique, the ampulla of Vater is identified endoscopically and a fine cannula inserted into the pancreatic duct. Small volumes of radio-opaque dye may then be injected to identify the pancreatic duct structure and any distortion or deformity within it. This technique is dangerous when pancreatic pseudocysts are present since they may become filled with dye and an abscess may be produced.

In the past, pancreatic angiography and pancreatic scintiscanning were used to identify structural abnormalities of the pancreas, but have now largely been superseded by pancreatic ultrasonography. In centres where the technique is available, whole body computerized tomography techniques are proving very valuable for the investigation of pancreatic structural abnormalities.

Gastroenterology department based investigations

In paediatric practice, sweat electrolyte investigations may be required for the diagnosis of cystic fibrosis, where the concentration of sodium in the sweat is elevated above 60 mmol per litre. The test is difficult to interpret in adult life. In the test, sweat is collected on a pad applied to the forearm in an area where sweat secretion has been stimulated by the application of heat and pilocarpine.

The exocrine function of the pancreas may be tested by stimulating pancreatic secretion and collecting pancreatic juice from the duodenum. These tests depend upon a skilled operator passing a tube into the stomach and duodenum under radiological control and thereafter collecting pancreatic juice after the stimulation of its flow by various alternative methods. The simplest method is to give a standard meal comprising carbohydrate, protein and fat called a Lundh meal. Alternatively, the pancreas may be stimulated by an intravenous injection of secretin. It is common to collect the stimulated pancreatic juice over a period of hours after which the laboratory will analyse the volume, bicarbonate and amylase concentrations. Alternatively ^{75}Se selenomethionine may be given intravenously since this istope concentrates in the pancreas. Any pancreatic juice stimulated by the above techniques is then radioactive and the concentration of radioactivity can be measured. Whichever of these techniques is chosen, a comparison with normal findings enables an evaluation of pancreatic function to be made. It is particularly useful to do these tests in the investigation of the cause of steatorrhoea.

The investigation of pancreatic exocrine function by the above tests using a tube technique are unpleasant and prolonged for the patient. Recent attempts have been made to provide a tubeless pancreatic function test in which pancreatic enzymes digest a chemical substance given by mouth and the products of digestion are subsequently absorbed. Their degradation products may be measured in the urine and an assessment made of the efficiency of pancreatic digestion. The tests of this type which are currently being evaluated are the urinary para-amino-benzoic acid test (PABA), the fluorescein dilaurate test and the cobalt isotope test. To date, none of these tests have been taken into routine use in the investigation of pancreatic pathology.

Endoscopic retrograde pancreatography is a useful investigation for the investigation of structural abnormalities of the pancreas. The performance of this test depends upon the Gastroenterology department and the Radiology department, since during the test radiographs of the structure of the pancreas will have to be taken. Apart from whole body computerized tomography, endoscopic retrograde pancreatography remains the sole method of producing radiological images of the pancreas and is useful in the identification of pancreatic neoplasm and parenchymal pancreatic disease. Overfilling of the pancreas with radio-opaque material is a hazard and may lead to secondary pancreatitis. Newer radio-opaque media are under development which may allow parenchymal filling of the pancreas with a greater degree of safety and may become very useful for identifying fine details of disturbance of pancreatic architecture.

NURSING CARE DURING INVESTIGATION

Sweat electrolyte test

Check list

Sweat electrolyte testing equipment
Weighed filter paper in container from Biochemistry laboratory
Lint squares
Water for washing area to be used
Cotton wool balls
Tissues
Pilocarpine (0.2% solution)
Magnesium sulphate (24.65 g in 1 litre distilled water)
Polythene
Waterproof strapping
Crepe bandages
Arrange for Biochemistry laboratory to process the sweat collection
Request form

Procedure

The procedure is explained to the parents of the child and consent obtained by the referring clinician. The arm to be used is washed with clean water and thoroughly dried. Two squares of lint are soaked in pilocarpine and placed on the flexural aspect of the arm. The positive electrode is placed on the lint and held in position. Two further squares of lint are soaked in magnesium sulphate and placed on the extensor aspect of the same arm. The negative electrode is placed on this lint and held in place, ensuring that the two lots of lint do not touch. The electrodes are now secured with the rubber bandage, tape or dry bandage.

The equipment is switched on and the rheostat slowly increased from the zero position to between 4 and 5 mA. Some tingling may be experienced but if the current increase is slow (over a period of 15–30 seconds) this can be avoided. The machine is left on for five minutes, the current being checked and adjusted as required.

After the procedure, the electrodes are removed and the forearm cleaned with water. The arm should then be thoroughly dried.

The area where the pilocarpine has been drawn into the skin will be slightly reddened. The filter paper is taken from the tube with forceps and placed on the reddened area. The filter paper should be kept in place by a clean strip of polythene which is fixed to the skin with waterproof tape, well-sealed around the edges. This is now covered with a crepe bandage. The patient resumes normal activities, leaving the filter paper in place for 30 minutes. At this stage, the filter paper should be inspected through the polythene to assess wetness and left in place for a further 30 minutes if necessary.

At the end of the test period, the paper is removed with forceps, returned to the container, labelled and despatched to the laboratory with a completed request form. The patient's arm is cleaned and dried ensuring that all waterproof strapping marks have been removed. The patient should be made happy and comfortable.

It is preferable, in order to obtain a reliable result, to perform two concurrent sweat tests.

Lundh test

Check list

12F single lumen weighted radio-opaque tube (e.g. Anderson AN20)
Lubricant
Gauze swabs
Adhesive tape
Large bowl with crushed ice

continued

Glass measuring flask for collection of secretions
30 ml syringe
Lundh meal
5 specimen containers for transporting collections to the laboratory
Request form
Arrange with laboratory to process the collections
Check 10-day rule if appropriate

Procedure

The patient should have fasted overnight. On receiving the patient, the nurse must ensure that the procedure is understood and informed written consent has been obtained by the referring clinician.

The patient is asked to clear the nose and the lubricated tube is passed pernasally. Radiological screening may be used to help locate the tube and ensure that it is positioned with the tip in the second part of the duodenum (Fig. 6.3).

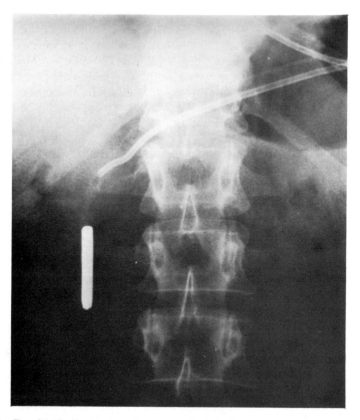

Fig. 6.3   Duodenal tube in place for pancreatic function test.

The duodenal juice is allowed to drain freely by siphonage into the flask sitting in the ice, approximately 80 cm below the level of the patient's head. Gentle suction with a syringe may be required periodically to ensure that good collections are obtained. When a substantial resting sample (10–20 ml) has been obtained, the stimulatory meal should be administered to the patient. Four consecutive half-hour samples of duodenal juice are then collected on ice. The five samples collected should be labelled carefully with the time obtained and stored in the deep freeze at −20°C until required for analysis. Appearance, volume and pH should be recorded prior to freezing of the samples.

On completion of the test, the tube should be removed and the patient made comfortable. Normal eating and drinking may commence.

Lundh test meal

The following formulation is the Lundh meal which is used in pancreatic function tests:

Ingredients: 18 g corn oil
15 g casein
40 mg glucose
made up in 300 ml water

Method: Mix casein and water first, then add glucose and corn oil. Blackcurrant juice or milk shake flavourings may be used to improve taste. An electric blender ensures adequate mixing of ingredients

Pancreatic function tests

Seleno-methionine (⁷⁵Se) test

Check list

Weighted sump tube e.g. Anderson AN20
or
Levin tube with mercury bag

Lubricant
Tissues
Adhesive tape
Gauze swabs
Disposable gloves for administrator of isotope
Lundh test meal
Check 10-day rule if appropriate, as this applies to both isotope administration and radiological screening
Arrange supply of ^{75}Se isotope in pre-loaded syringe from Isotope laboratory and liaise with the laboratory for subsequent analysis of samples
Arrange radiological screening facilities for placement of tube

Procedure

The patient arrives after an overnight fast. On receiving the patient, the nurse ensures that the procedure is understood and informed written consent has been obtained by the referring clinician. Reassurance is necessary as the patient may find the intubation unpleasant and intolerance of the tube is common. The patient should be weighed before intubation commences. If possible the patient should sit upright in a comfortable chair or on a bed and asked to clear the nose. The tube is lubricated and passed via the nose or the mouth. Radiological screening is necessary to ensure that the tip of the tube is located in the second part of the duodenum.

When the tube is in a satisfactory position, the test meal is given orally and must be taken in its entirety. It can be taken via a straw if preferred. The isotope is given intravenously ten minutes later. Gloves should be worn when handling the isotope and care is necessary to ensure that all of the isotope is given by use of barbotage. This involves withdrawing sufficient venous blood to rinse the syringe and the needle 'dead space' and reinjecting this blood.

The patient is allowed to rest comfortably in the right lateral position with the tube closed off for two hours. Duodenal juice is then aspirated and a collection of 10–20 ml obtained either by syringe or by siphonage directly into a container. The aliquot should be labelled and sent to the laboratory for analysis with a completed request form. The syringe and needle with which the isotope has been administered should be returned to the Isotope laboratory for disposal. The patient is made comfortable and allowed to eat and drink normally.

This is an unpleasant investigation and requires skilled nursing care in order to achieve a satisfactory result. Metoclopramide should be avoided as this will stimulate duodenal activity and cause secretions to be lost in the digestive tract. Sedation may be given to the very distressed patient.

Secretin pancreatic function test

Check list

Double lumen duodenal tube e.g. Dreiling type
Lubricant
Gauze swabs
Adhesive tape
Two suction pumps suitable for continuous suction of body cavities
Crushed ice in bowl large enough to hold flask of one suction pump
20 ml syringes to aspirate duodenal secretions
Containers for collected secretions
Stimulant – secretin
Saline for mixing stimulant
Syringes – 2 ml and 5 ml for administration of stimulant
Needles for i.v. injections

continued

Stop watch or time clock
Arrange radiological screening for placement of tube
Check 10-day rule if appropriate
This procedure should be arranged in advance with the laboratory to ensure satisfactory co-operation and results

---

Procedure

The patient arrives after an overnight fast. On receiving the patient, the nurse ensures that the procedure has been understood and informed written consent has been obtained by the referring clinician. Reassurance is necessary as the patient may find the intubation unpleasant and intolerance of the tube is common. The patient should be weighed prior to intubation. The patient is allowed to sit in a comfortable position in a chair or on a bed and the tube is passed orally. It may be necessary to use an introducing wire to help pass the tube and this can be especially helpful when the distal tip reaches the pylorus.

The tube is positioned under radiological control. The double lumen tube is required to separate gastric and duodenal secretions to prevent dilution and neutralization of the alkaline pancreatic excretions. The tube is therefore positioned with the distal tip and holes in the second part of the duodenum and the proximal holes lying on the greater curve of the stomach. The sections of the tube can easily be visualized radiologically.

The patient is positioned comfortably in the left lateral position and the proximal ends of the double lumen tube are connected to the aspiration pumps. The tube labelled 'gastric lumen' is left at a pressure of 4–5 mm Hg. The tube labelled 'duodenal lumen' is also maintained at a pressure of 4–5 mm Hg and the glass flask of this pump is positioned in a bowl of crushed ice. The ice helps to keep the secretions in a stable condition prior to analysis.

Residual duodenal contents should be aspirated and discarded. Secretin, 1–2 units per kg body weight, is now given intravenously and duodenal juice collected and the volume measured every 10 minutes for one hour. The collections should be stored in a refrigerator.

The samples are measured for total volume and correctly labelled prior to prompt transport from the refrigerator to the laboratory, with the completed request form. Laboratory analysis for bicarbonate, trypsin and amylase content can be undertaken.

On completion of the test, the tube is removed, the patient made comfortable and allowed to eat and drink normally.

This is an unpleasant investigation and requires skilled nursing care in order to achieve a satisfactory result. Metoclopramide should be avoided as this will stimulate duodenal activity and cause secretions to be lost in the digestive tract. Sedation may be given to the distressed patient.

N-Benzoyl-C-tyrosyl-p-aminobenzoic acid (B-T PABA) pancreatic function test

In this test, the patient receives an oral pancreatic stimulant and an isotope. Urinalysis is used to ascertain pancreatic function, thereby making this a more acceptable and simpler form of investigation.

Check list

Test meal: 25 g casein

300 ml water

Flavouring – blackcurrant juice or milk shake flavouring

Isotope ^{14}C PABA, the dose having been pre-determined by the Isotope laboratory

B-T PABA as prescribed by the clinician

Protective gloves for nurse and patient

Jug and funnel for urine collection – individually labelled for each patient

6 hour collection container

2×20 ml containers for aliquots

Arrange provision of isotope with Isotope laboratory and the subsequent analysis of urine samples

---

Procedure

The patient arrives after an overnight fast, having avoided prunes, cranberries, anchovies, paracetamol and alcohol for 48 hours. On receiving the patient, the nurse ensures that the procedure is understood and that informed written consent has been obtained by the referring clinician. A 20 ml aliquot of heparinized blood may be taken for biochemical screening.

The patient is asked to empty the bladder and a 20 ml aliquot of urine is saved in a labelled container. The mixed test meal including both isotope and B-T PABA is now given to the patient who may now drink free fluids for 6 hours and collect all urine in the container provided. Protective gloves should be worn by the patient when collecting the urine. The patient should be made comfortable with easy access to toilet facilities. It is possible for the patient to complete this test at home. The total volume of urine passed in the six-hour period is measured and from it a further 20 ml aliquot is collected in a labelled container. Both aliquots are sent to the laboratory with the completed request form. All remaining urine is discarded and collecting equipment rinsed under running cold water before disposal. The patient may now eat and drink normally and resume any medication regime.

Endoscopic retrograde pancreatography (Fig. 6.4)

This procedure is managed in the same way as endoscopic retrograde cholangiography with some additional requirements.

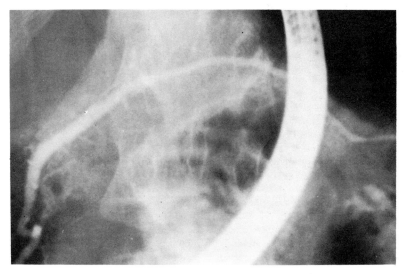

Fig. 6.4   *Endoscopic retrograde pancreatogram (ERP).*

Check list

As for endoscopic retrograde cholangiography, p. 151, plus:

Foam wedges or other positioning aids to ensure that all of the pancreas is visualized easily during the procedure by correct positioning of the patient

10 ml syringes − these should be large enough to fill the cannulae and ducts as overfilling can cause discomfort to the patient and a rise in serum amylase after the procedure. It is possible to completely fill the pancreatic duct with only 4−5 ml of contrast

Complications

These are as for endoscopic retrograde cholangiography and sphincterotomy.

7

THE LARGE INTESTINE

ANATOMY

The large intestine runs from the ileocaecal valve to the anus. In sequence, from the ileocaecal valve distally it is subdivided into the caecum, ascending colon, transverse colon, descending colon, sigmoid colon, rectum and anus.

The caecum lies in the right iliac fossa and the terminal ileum enters it from the side through the ileocaecal valve. The appendix is attached to the base of the caecum. From the caecum, the ascending colon runs on the right side of the abdomen to the underside of the liver where it turns towards the mid-line round a bend called the hepatic flexure to become the transverse colon. This loops across the front of the abdomen below the level of the stomach to reach the underside of the diaphragm on the left-hand side of the abdomen close to the hilum of the spleen. At this level, the colon turns downwards round the splenic flexure to become the descending colon which ends in the left iliac fossa to form the sigmoid colon. The sigmoid colon runs into the pelvis and ends in the capacious, tortuous rectum which is characterized internally by prominent mucosal folds called the valves of Houston. The rectum terminates at the anus where there are strong circular muscle bands called the internal and external sphincters.

As elsewhere, the colonic portion of the intestine comprises mucosal, submucosal, muscular and serosal layers. In the colon, however, the longitudinal muscle layers are gathered together into three broad bands called taeniae which pucker the colon into its characteristic folds or haustrae. The circular muscle coats are also well developed. The blood supply of the right side of the colon is derived from arterial arcades which are supplied by the superior mesenteric artery, whilst the left side of the colon including the sigmoid is supplied by the inferior mesenteric artery (Fig. 7.1).

PHYSIOLOGY

The colon has one main function. In transporting waste material from the alimentary canal out of the body, fluid is absorbed from the waste material

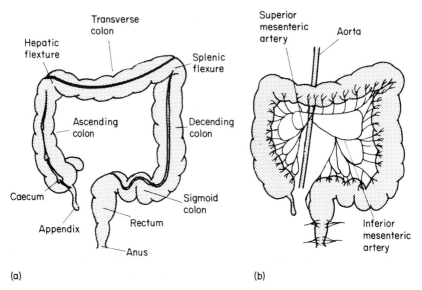

Fig. 7.1   *Anatomy and blood supply of large intestine. (a) General structure, (b) arterial arcades.*

thus conserving the body's water and giving faeces a suitable consistency for evacuation. Under normal circumstances, the progressively more solid faeces are propelled along the colon by peristaltic waves. This passage of faeces through the colon may be accelerated when the activity of the muscles is increased. This may occur during infections of the colon or during disease involvement. The passage of faeces along the colon with reabsorption of water is a process which takes place under the influence of the autonomic nervous system.

Once faeces reach the rectum, distension of this part of the large bowel prompts a desire to defaecate through reflex mechanisms. These reflex actions can be voluntarily inhibited such that the desire to defaecate passes away. Long-term inhibition of the desire to defaecate may lead to chronic constipation so that evacuation may occur only at intervals of weeks or months and may require increasing amounts of purgatives to empty the rectum and colon. This is particularly common in elderly people or in the sick and debilitated. Any inflammation of the mucosa of the colon reduces water absorption and leads to diarrhoea. In addition, chronic inflammation of the mucosa results in the production of an excessive amount of mucus which may be passed with the stools and may be apparent to the patient.

PATHOLOGY (Fig. 7.2)

Ulcerative colitis

The aetiology of ulcerative colitis is unknown. Like Crohn's disease it may be due to an abnormal immune response either to infection or to food products.

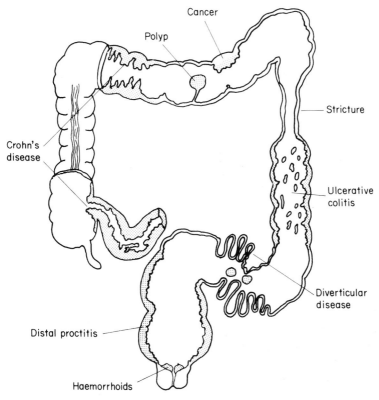

Fig. 7.2 *Important disorders of the large intestine.*

In a few patients, withdrawal of milk from the diet improves symptoms, suggesting an allergy to milk protein. There is a familial tendency and an association within family groups between ulcerative colitis, ankylosing spondylitis and Crohn's disease. It has been suggested that psychological factors may predispose to the condition but it seems more likely that personality disorders are generated by symptoms of the disease rather than vice versa. The inflammatory process may be limited to the rectum (distal proctitis), involve the descending colon (proctocolitis) or involve the whole colon as far as the caecum (total colitis). Occasionally, the terminal ileum may seem to be involved (backwash ileitis). Characteristically, whatever the extent of the disease, the mucosal change is continuous throughout the affected area in contrast to the patchy changes of Crohn's disease. In the mild form, the mucosa is oedematous and reddened with a slightly granular change and a tendency to punctate haemorrhage and contact bleeding during investigative procedures. In more severe involvement, ulceration of the mucosa develops in which the ulcers may be superficial or penetrate deeply into the mucosa, sometimes undermining it. In very severe cases the mucosal lining of the large bowel may slough completely.

Sometimes, regenerative islands of comparatively normal mucosa produce polypoid change (pseudopolyposis). In acute disease, the colon may become greatly dilated with an extremely thin wall which may actually perforate (toxic dilatation of the colon). In chronic, long-standing cases, the colon becomes shortened, narrowed and featureless with a lack of haustral markings.

Microscopically, inflammation is confined to the mucosa where oedema, intramucosal haemorrhage and inflammatory cell infiltrate can readily be identified. The number of mucus-producing goblet cells is reduced and collections of polymorphs appear in the mucosa, so-called 'crypt abscesses'.

The disease may occur at all ages but like Crohn's disease, is commonest between the ages of 20 and 40 years. The hallmark of the condition is recurrent attacks of bloody diarrhoea. If severe, the attacks may lead to dehydration or the sinister complication of toxic dilatation of the colon with tachycardia, high pyrexia and abdominal distension. In the course of this complication perforation of the colon may occur. When the disease is confined to the rectum (distal proctitis), the symptoms are usually mild and consist simply of loose motions with increased mucus and blood-streaking of the stools. Even short segment disease of this nature, however, may cause severely debilitating diarrhoea, urgency of defaecation and bleeding. Usually, systemic disturbance is absent and the complication of toxic dilatation not observed. It is rare for distal proctitis to spread more proximally and develop into left-sided or total colonic disease. The diagnosis may be suspected from the history and confirmed by sigmoidoscopic inspection of the rectum supported by the histological evidence obtained from rectal biopsy. Whilst this inspection will confirm the nature of the disease, the full extent of the process can only be assessed by performing a barium enema. It is dangerous to perform barium enema during severe attacks of ulcerative colitis, since there is some evidence that toxic dilatation may be precipitated by doing so. In severe cases, plain abdominal radiography may often indicate the extent of the disease process, since the colon will usually contain enough air to outline the abnormal mucosal pattern.

Bacteriological studies should be performed to exclude bacillary and amoebic dysentery and tuberculous enterocolitis where appropriate. The radiological features of the disease are usually sufficient to differentiate it from Crohn's disease which may also affect the colon (Table 7.1).

In some cases, radiology and rigid sigmoidoscopy are inadequate to accurately assess the true nature and extent of the disease. Under these circumstances, fibreoptic colonoscopy is valuable since the true nature of mucosal involvement can be identified and multiple biopsies may be taken. Since chronic ulcerative colitis carries a risk of malignancy in the long term, colonoscopic inspection with multiple biopsies might prove of benefit in detecting early malignant change. Colonoscopy should not be performed in the severely ill patient since there is a risk of colonic perforation or massive bacteraemia in these circumstances.

Table 7.1   Radiological differentation between Crohn's disease and ulcerative colitis

Factors favouring Crohn's disease
Small bowel involvement
Rectal sparing
Discontinuous disease
Predominantly right-sided colonic involvement
Asymmetrical loss of haustrations
Deep fissuring
Longitudinal fissuring

Crohn's disease of the colon

Chronic inflammation of the colon may occur in Crohn's disease. The condition may mimic ulcerative colitis, with recurrent attacks of abdominal pain, colic, urgency of defaecation and diarrhoea. There is usually less rectal bleeding. Characteristically, Crohn's colitis usually affects the right side of the colon more than the left and the rectum is often spared, unlike ulcerative colitis where the reverse is the case. Perianal disease with prominent skin tags, fissures and fistulae is much more common in Crohn's colitis.

The investigation of this condition is identical to that of ulcerative colitis from which it must be differentiated. Once the diagnosis of Crohn's colitis has been established, it is important to exclude small bowel involvement by performing a barium follow-through study of the small intestine.

Diverticular disease

The presence of saccular outpouchings from the colonic wall is known as diverticulosis. Sometimes the pockets become inflamed when the condition is known as diverticulitis. The two phases of this disorder are known collectively as diverticular disease. It is not known why diverticula form, but it is probable that abnormal pressure patterns within the lumen of the colon push out mucosal pockets through defects in the muscle layers. As a result, the saccular projections consist of mucosa and serosa only and contain no muscular component. It is probable that abnormal pressure patterns within the colonic lumen are the result of dietary factors. It is known that diverticular disease is rare in areas of the world where the diet has a high fibre content. On the other hand, the disease is increasing in Western countries where refined foods are consumed which contain less natural fibre. Experimental work has shown that intra-colonic pressures vary with the bulk of faecal residue and high faecal weight is associated with low intraluminal pressures. Diverticular disease is most common in middle and late adult life and affects males and females equally.

The sigmoid colon is the commonest area to be involved. The muscle wall is greatly thickened, in which thin-walled pockets can be readily identified. Many of them contain small, hard pellets of faeces called faecoliths. When present, inflammation may lead to local abscess formation, fistulae or even peritonitis. With repeated attacks of inflammation, the bowel wall becomes progressively thickened with narrowing of the lumen and features of partial colonic obstruction. Although the commonest site of involvement is in the sigmoid colon, diverticula may occur at any site and may be so extensive as to involve the total length of the colon.

Patients most frequently complain of pain in the left iliac fossa with abdominal distension, local tenderness and altered bowel habit. Occasionally, rectal bleeding may occur with infrequent episodes of fever and features suggestive of peritonitis and intestinal obstruction. Because of pressure of an inflamed segment of diverticular disease upon the bladder, symptoms of frequency and dysuria may suggest a urinary infection. Very rarely, a fistula may develop between colon and bladder whereupon faecal matter may be present in the urine. A barium enema is necessary to assess the extent of the diverticular disease and severity of the disorder. Sigmoidoscopy is necessary to exclude a cancer in the rectum or sigmoid colon which might mimic diverticular disease and to exclude the remote possibility of co-existent cancer. If diverticular narrowing is identified in a more proximal segment then colonoscopy may be required for the same purpose.

Cancer of the colon and rectum

In the Western world, cancer of the large intestine is the commonest malignancy of the gastrointestinal tract. Since the disorder is rare in Africa and Asia, speculation has arisen that dietary factors or differences in bacterial flora may play a part in aetiology. Long-standing ulcerative colitis and familial multiple polyposis of the colon are pre-malignant conditions. Two-thirds of cancers of the large bowel occur in the left colon or rectum. Between 2 and 5% of colon cancers have a synchronous lesion in another part of the colon. If multiple polyps are present this figure may reach 10%. On gross inspection, either by colonoscopy or directly at operation, the tumours are most frequently proliferative, fungating and ulcerated. Local structures may be infiltrated including the bowel wall whilst polypoidal tumours or annular strictures may also arise. Secondary spread is via lymphatics and the bloodstream to both local and distant sites, especially the liver.

Symptoms vary, dependent upon the site of the cancer. The most common presenting features are of rectal bleeding, altered bowel habit and abdominal pain. Cancers of the left side of the colon commonly present early with features of colonic obstruction. On the other hand, cancers of the right side of the colon often present late so that severe anaemia and general systemic upset are more common. If the tumour is in the lower sigmoid or rectum then urgency of defaecation and feeling of incomplete emptying of the rectum may be present. Examination of the patient may not be very helpful but digital rectal examination must always be performed. Inspection of the stools for obvious blood or tests for the presence of occult blood should be undertaken. Investigation includes the performance of a standard barium enema, but superficial and small cancers can be missed by this technique, and a special modification called a double-contrast barium enema gives better results. Here, smaller amounts of barium followed by air are introduced into the colon to give lighter mucosal coating. By doing this, even small cancers can be detected. In cases where a barium enema has raised the suspicion of a cancer beyond the reach of the sigmoidoscope then colonoscopy is essential. Even if the malignancy is only suspected, a biopsy can usually be obtained to establish the diagnosis.

Benign tumours of the large intestine

Colonic polyps are fairly common. They may be single or multiple and are most commonly found in the left side of the colon. They may be sessile, which means that they have a broad base across the normal colonic mucosa, or pedunculated which indicates that they have a stalk. In this latter case, the stalk may allow the polyp to move up and down the lumen of the bowel. These benign tumours may be found coincidentally at barium enema, colonoscopy, or at operation. They may present with recurrent rectal bleeding, increased mucus in the stools or recurrent vague abdominal pain. Whilst primarily benign, evidence is accumulating that colon cancer most commonly arises in pre-existing colon polyps and that the size of the polyp is important. Any polyp greater than 1.0 cm in diameter should be regarded as pre-malignant (Fig. 7.3). Most polyps up to this size and often those of a larger size may be removed at colonoscopy using a diathermy technique. In the condition called familial multiple polyposis of the colon, the disorder runs in families and there may be thousands of small polyps on the surface of the colon and rectum. Whilst initially benign, these polyps always become malignant in due course. The only way to prevent this is to undertake total colectomy in early adult life.

Ischaemic colitis

Occlusion of the inferior mesenteric artery will lead to ischaemia of the left colon. This disorder is termed ischaemic colitis. The effects upon the colon may vary depending on the severity of the arterial insufficiency and upon its acuteness. In the most severe cases, a short segment of the colon may become

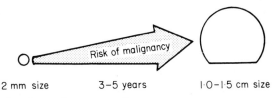

| 2 mm size | 3–5 years | 1·0–1·5 cm size |

Fig. 7.3 *The little polyp–adenoma–malignancy sequence.*

gangrenous and perforate. When less severe, ulceration and bleeding from the colonic mucosa may occur. In chronic low grade ischaemia, gradual stricturing of the colon may occur, most commonly in the region of the splenic flexure. Stricture formation may also be the end-result of a moderate to severe acute episode. Since patients present with abdominal pain, bloody diarrhoea or even a radiologically identified stricture, the importance of ischaemic colitis lies in differentiating the disorder from conditions which it may mimic such as carcinoma, ulcerative colitis or diverticular disease. Direct colonoscopic inspection and mucosal biopsies will aid differentiation from these other disorders.

Recurrent haemorrhage from the colon

Haemorrhoids are the commonest cause of rectal bleeding. These prominent veins in the anal canal characteristically produce jets of bright red blood at the time of defaecation. Bright red blood may also be seen on the toilet tissue at the end of defaecation. When blood arises from disorders higher in the colon, then it may present as clots or as darkly altered blood or melaena. Some lesions do not bleed enough to cause obvious blood in the stools, but it may be detected by chemical means. Although these patients may not have obvious rectal blood loss, the continuing low grade loss may be sufficient to produce anaemia.

Angiodysplasia of the colon is a rare disorder occurring especially in the elderly and mainly affecting the right side of the colon. Vascular malformations within the mucosa can bleed intermittently. Sometimes the bleeding may be profuse. Rectal examination, barium enema and sigmoidoscopy will usually be necessary to identify the cause of rectal bleeding, but if the cause is not identified by these means, and colonoscopy and angiography may both be necessary. This is usually the only way that angiodysplasia can be detected. Diathermic removal of polyps or ablation of angiodysplastic lesions is possible through the colonoscope.

Causes of high colonic bleeding are given in Table 7.2.

Table 7.2   The causes of high colonic bleeding

Ulcerative colitis and Crohn's disease
Cancer of the colon
Colonic polyps
Ischaemic colitis
Diverticular disease
Angiodysplasia of the colonic mucosa

Irritable bowel syndrome

One of the commonest disorders of the alimentary tract is long-standing abdominal pain with altered bowel habit for which no cause can be found.

This symptom cluster is known as the irritable bowel syndrome or spastic colon. Although benign, its importance lies in its ability to mimic more sinister colonic pathology. Several factors may be involved in its causation. There is no doubt that psychological disturbances are frequent, and sufferers are often tense, anxious individuals who worry excessively about the problems of life. Alternatively, many patients may relate the onset of their symptoms to an episode of infective diarrhoea or even to a course of antibiotics for another condition. The syndrome occurs most frequently in women, usually between the ages of 20 and 40 years. The symptom complex consists of constipation or painless diarrhoea, or alternating phases of both. Recurrent attacks of abdominal pain are commonplace. The pain may be of a continuous dull aching quality or sometimes colicky. Defaecation often improves the pain whilst it is sometimes provoked by food. Other symptoms include abdominal distension, an awareness of intestinal action with prominent bowel sounds and recurrent attacks of nausea. Associated tiredness and weakness may occur. Patients frequently complain of associated symptoms such as migraine, urinary symptoms, painful menses and pelvic pain during sexual intercourse. Despite the severity of the symptoms, comprehensive investigation of the gastrointestinal tract fails to identify an organic cause for the symptoms although increased muscular activity in the colon is commonly observed. One of the problems of the disorder is that its symptoms may mimic many other disorders so that comprehensive investigation is necessary to exclude more treatable conditions.

Infections of the colon

The commonest infections which affect the colon and cause diarrhoea are bacillary dysentery caused by the organism *Shigella sonnei* and by various species of *Salmonella*. Diarrhoea is usually short-lived, but may cause severe debility, especially in the frail and elderly patient. Amoebic dysentery on the other hand, is caused by infection with a parasite called *Entamoeba histolytica*. Cysts of the parasite survive well outside the body and are ingested in water or uncooked food which has been contaminated by human faeces. Once absorbed, the active form emerges from the cysts in the colon and whilst they remain free in the colon, the condition is asymptomatic. Under certain circumstances, invasion and ulceration of the mucus membrane of the large bowel takes place, thus causing the symptoms of amoebic dysentery. Characteristically, flask-shaped ulcers may be identified surrounded by healthy looking mucosa. Rarely, parasites may pass to the liver and produce an amoebic abscess, or a localized granuloma may occur in the colon. The diagnosis may be established by finding cysts or parasites in the stools and identifying the flask-shaped ulcers on direct sigmoidoscopic inspection.

Schistosomiasis, whilst rare in the Western world is an important cause of colonic disease in the tropics, where it may be spread by faecal contamination of irrigation systems. The most important aspect of involvement in the colon is of recurrent rectal bleeding, polypoid formation and fibrous strictures. The rectum is most commonly affected, but the whole colon may become involved. Localized stricture formation may occur which must be differentiated from malignant change.

In patients who have received prolonged courses of antibiotics, pseudomembranous colitis may occur and result in diarrhoea. Unless the offending antibiotic is withdrawn, symptoms may persist and may become so severe that death may ensue. This disorder has now been recognized as being due to colonization of the colon with an organism called *Clostridium difficile*. It is extremely difficult to grow this organism from colonic contents but the toxin produced can be readily identified. Once confirmed, the condition usually responds to withdrawal of the offending antibiotic and treatment with a course of vancomycin. Detection of the *C. difficile* toxin in the stool is sufficient confirmation of the diagnosis but the pseudomembrane can be seen sigmoidoscopically and its presence can be confirmed histologically.

INVESTIGATION OF DISEASES OF THE LARGE INTESTINE

Laboratory based tests:
  Blood: Routine haematology: Haemoglobin, full blood count, sedimentation rate
      Serum biochemical tests: Serum electrolytes and blood urea
                Serum liver function tests
                Serum orosomucoid or mucoprotein
      Serum agglutination and complement fixation tests for infecting agents
  Stool: Microscopy for parasites
       Culture for bacteria
       Analysis for faecal occult blood
Radiology:
  Standard barium enema
  Double-contrast barium enema
  Angiography
Gastroenterology department procedures:
  Proctoscopy
  Sigmoidoscopy
  Fibreoptic sigmoidoscopy
  Colonoscopy
  Mucosal biopsy at any level
  Colonic polypectomy
  Diathermy of bleeding lesions

Conventional radiology

Barium enema is the commonest investigation of this type. The procedure is uncomfortable and often exhausting particularly for the elderly patient in whom cardiac disease or arrhythmias may be present. The barium enema should always be preceded by proper examination of the abdomen and by digital rectal examination and by sigmoidoscopy. The technique requires the introduction of barium alone, or barium and air, into the rectum through a balloon catheter. The radiologist then manipulates the patient into various positions to obtain good views of the total colon. The best mucosal pictures are produced when a double-contrast technique is used. In this, less barium is introduced and air is used to coat the small amount of barium onto the mucosal surface of the colon. At a late stage in the inspection, the patient empties the colon of as much barium as possible and these emptying or post-evacuation films give valuable additional information. It is important to remember that inadvertent irradiation in the first few weeks of pregnancy may lead to foetal damage which may be responsible for deformity or still-birth. In general therefore, women of child-bearing age should only have radiology in the ten days immediately following the onset of the last menstrual period (Fig. 7.4).

Endoscopy

Proctoscopy and rigid sigmoidoscopy are simple procedures which should always be carried out in patients with symptoms referable to the lower colon or rectum. It is commonplace to carry out these procedures without preparation in an outpatient clinic, but if the rectum contains faeces, then the procedure should be repeated after prior preparation with suppositories or an evacuation enema. Using these rigid instruments the lower 20 cm of the large bowel can usually be inspected.

Higher parts of the colon can be inspected with fibreoptic instruments. These vary in length from 60–180 cm and with them either the left side of the colon or total colonoscopy can be performed. The major benefits of these procedures are reasonable comfort for the patient and an ability to obtain excellent mucosal views. Biopsies may be obtained of any lesion identified and an additional benefit is the ability to remove polyps with a diathermy snare.

Stool examination

Simple inspection of the stool may provide important information with regard to the presence of blood or parasites. Culture of the stool may identify pathogens such as *Shigella sonnei*, whilst direct microscopic inspection of the stools is of value in distinguishing amoebic dysentery from other disorders. Tests for occult blood may be of value in patients with recurrent or persistent anaemia in whom obvious blood loss through the rectum has not been identified.

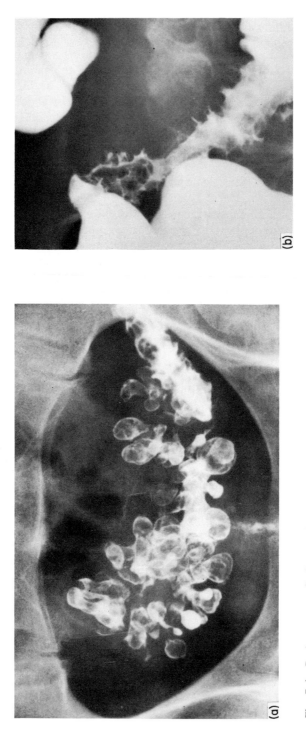

Fig. 7.4 *Barium enema findings in large bowel disease. (a) Diverticular disease, (b) Crohn's colitis.*

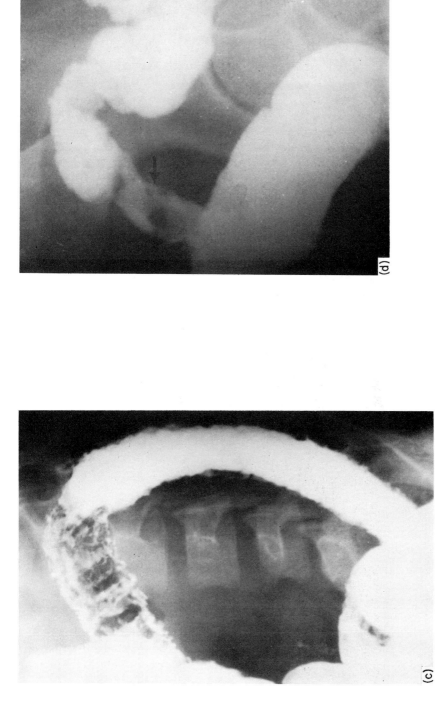

Fig. 7.4 (c) Ulcerative colitis and (d) carcinoma sigmoid colon.

(c)

(d)

BOWEL PREPARATION PRIOR TO ENDOSCOPIC EXAMINATION OF THE LARGE INTESTINE

Sigmoidoscopy and proctoscopy

Glycerine suppositories (see patient instructions in Appendix B)

Fibresigmoidoscopy

Glycerine suppositories (see patient instructions in Appendix B)
Phosphate enema
Oxyphenisatin (Veripaque 3 g in 1500 ml warm water)

Colonoscopy

Dietary restrictions (see Appendix B)
Purgatives: Senna preparations (see letter to patient in Appendix B)
          Sodium picosulphate (see letter to patient in Appendix B)
Oral 10% mannitol
Colonic lavage
Herculean preparation

Administration of enemas

Check list

Enemas of choice
Jug/bowl of hot water, to heat enemas to body temperature
Disposable gloves
Gauze swabs
Lubricant
Incontinence pad
Tissues
Bed pan/easy access to toilet facilities
Screens
Air deodorizer

Procedure

The patient is positioned in the left lateral position. The tube of the bag containing the enema is lubricated and gently inserted into the rectum. With even pressure, the enema is expelled into the rectum and the patient is asked to hold the fluid for up to 20 minutes if possible. The lower end of the bed or couch may be elevated to make this easier. Convenient access to toilet facilities or provision of a bed pan are important. Two enemas may be administered if required. It should be remembered that phosphate enemas give poor results in the presence of diverticular disease, stricturing or ileorectal anastomosis.

In certain situations enemas may be self-administered, in which case full instructions must be provided.

Oral 10% mannitol

Before preparation of the bowel with 10% mannitol, dietary restrictions should be observed (see Appendix B).

On arrival the patient is given 20 mg metoclopramide (Maxolon) orally. Thirty minutes later the patient is asked to drink 1 litre of a cold solution containing 100 g mannitol, as rapidly as possible, normally within half an hour.

Thereafter, water in as large a quantity as possible should be drunk and a mouthwash or mints given as required for mouth dryness. The patient is also given castor oil/zinc barrier cream to apply to the anus to avoid soreness from diarrhoea.

Colonoscopy is performed not less than three hours after mannitol ingestion. All patients are carefully observed to ensure that dehydration does not occur.

The only practical difficulty with this method of bowel preparation is that 300–400 ml of fluid may be left in the colon, requiring aspiration by the endoscopist. If mannitol is used, carbon dioxide exchange with the colon gas is required when diathermy is used as there is a risk of explosion due to increased levels of hydrogen and methane in the bowel.

Colonic lavage using the Henderson Lavage Machine

Check list

Henderson Lavage Machine filled to required volume (up to 12.5 litres (22 pints)) with warm water by mixing the hot and cold supply (Fig. 7.5)
Rectal nozzle (adult or paediatric) sterilized
Lubricant
Gauze swabs
Tissues

Procedure

The patient is positioned comfortably on a couch and kept warm during the procedure. Ensure that the temperature of the fluid in the machine is registering at 36°C on the thermometer on the front of the case.

Connect the tubing from the machine firmly over the connection marked 'inflow attachment' and the other end to the appropriate connection on the rectal nozzle. Repeat this procedure for the outflow attachment.

Lubricate the rectal nozzle and gently insert into the patient's rectum. Turn the inflow lever on and water will flow into the patient and return through the outflow tubing to the machine. Approximately 0.85 litres (1.5 pints) will be required to prime the circuit and the colon will generally accept up to 1.1 litres (2 pints).

Careful observation of the water level gauge is required in conjunction with

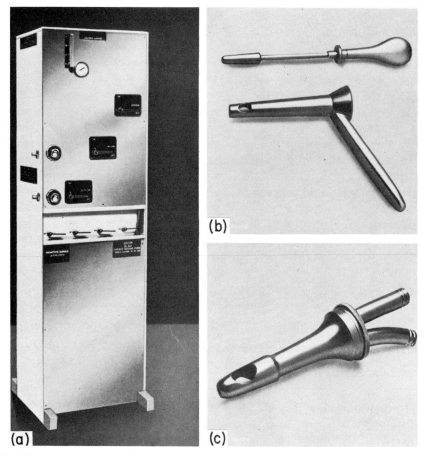

Fig. 7.5   *Components of the Henderson Lavage System. (a) Machine, (b) child nozzle, and (c) adult nozzle. (Courtesy of Macarthys Surgical Ltd.)*

patient observation during the filling routine. It is important to avoid over-filling of the colon.

After 1.1 litres (2 pints) have been introduced into the colon, the inflow lever is turned off and the vacuum started by turning the syphon lever on. Evacuation is achieved by switching the outflow lever to 'on'. The outflow can be observed through the outflow indication glass. When the turbulence stops the bowel has been emptied. The outflow lever can then be switched off and the cycle repeated until the outflow water is clear.

It is important that patients being prepared for colonoscopy this way are given dietary instructions and purgative preparations in the previous 48 hours.

Care of the Henderson Lavage Machine

The internal tank should be emptied by means of the drain tap. This is then closed along with all other taps and levers.

The internal tank lid is then opened and the air bleed valve turned off. The inflow and outflow are connected with tubing to the appropriate patient tubing attachments. The outflow lever and the purge lever are then turned on.

To prepare the machine for use, the purge lever and the outflow lever are turned off, the tubing disconnected and the air bleed valve turned on.

Herculean preparation

In this method of bowel preparation, the lavage is administered via a nasogastric tube. This is positioned in the stomach under radiological control and the patient is seated in a special toilet cabinet, on a cushioned lavatory seat.

The irrigant consists of:

Isotonic saline, sodium chloride (6.14 g)
Potassium chloride (0.75 g)
Sodium bicarbonate (2.94 g)
Distilled water (1000 ml)

and is warmed to 37°C and delivered through the stomach tube at 75 ml per min by a regulatory pump.

The first bowel motion is usually passed 40–60 min from the start of irrigation; clear fluid may be passed after 90 min and irrigation can be continued for another hour. Total irrigation time is 2–3 h and may involve 9–12 litres of irrigant. This method of preparation requires careful medical and nursing supervision and is not advisable in the elderly patient.

Complications of bowel preparations

These are nausea, vomiting electrolyte imbalance and syncope. Careful observation of all patients is necessary.

CARE OF THE PATIENT DURING GASTROENTEROLOGY-BASED INVESTIGATIONS AND THERAPEUTIC PROCEDURES

Sigmoidoscopy and proctoscopy

Check list

Proctoscope: with obturator (Fig. 7.6)
Sigmoidoscope: with obturator
                flex
                light source
                bellows
Lubricant
Gauze swabs
Tissues

continued

Disposable gloves
Biopsy forceps
Suction tube
Suction apparatus
Container and form for histology specimen

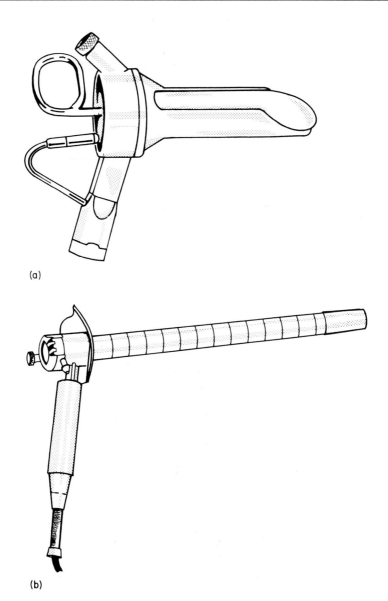

(a)

(b)

Fig. 7.6   *(a) Proctoscope and (b) rigid sigmoidoscope 25 cm in length.*

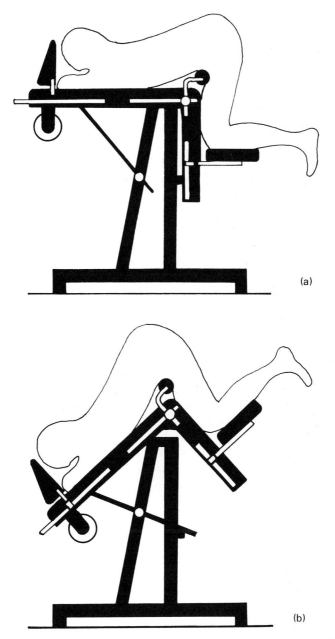

(a)

(b)

Fig. 7.7 *A purpose-built tilting couch for use in sigmoidoscopy conducted in the knee-elbow position.*

Procedure

To prepare the rectum and sigmoid colon for inspection, the patient will receive two glycerine suppositories before the examination. These should be inserted as far as possible into the rectum either by the ward or department nurse and an interval of 1–2 hours allowed to elapse before sigmoidoscopy. If the patient is at home, the suppositories may be sent with the appointment letter and the patient asked to self-administer them. Clear instructions must be sent to the patient to ensure that self-administration is carried out correctly (see Appendix B). If the patient is elderly or unable to read and understand these instructions, it will be necessary for the nurse to administer the suppositories in the department prior to the examination.

It is unnecessary for the patient to fast before this procedure. On arrival, the nurse ensures that the procedure is understood by the patient and informed written consent obtained by the referring clinician. Underwear below the waist should be removed and the patient given protective hospital clothing.

The patient is positioned either in the left lateral position on a trolley or in the knee–elbow position on a purpose-designed examination table (Fig. 7.7). The nurse must maintain the patient in the correct position during the examination as any involuntary movement may cause mucosal damage. After digital examination, the sigmoidoscope is inserted with the obturator in place.

Examination of the rectum and sigmoid colon up to 25 cm from the anus is possible in a patient with a well-prepared bowel and in whom the correct examining position is maintained. Mucosal biopsies may be obtained during this procedure. These will usually be obtained from below 15 cm in the rectum as this is below the peritoneal reflection and lessens the risk of perforation in the event of a full thickness biopsy.

At the end of the procedure, the patient is made clean and comfortable. Any biopsy specimens are mounted on card and transferred to the Histology laboratory in the correct container accompanied by a completed request form.

If required, limited rectal examination using a shorter proctoscope may be performed. The preparation and nursing procedure for this is identical to sigmoidoscopy.

Fibresigmoidoscopy

Check list

Fibreoptic sigmoidoscope
Light source
Suction pump
Accessories: cleaning brush
            biopsy forceps
            diathermy equipment

continued

Drugs: Buscopan ⎤
      pethidine ⎬ according to the clinician's requirements and the
      Buscopan ⎦ patient's needs
Container for biopsy
Histology request form

Procedure

On arrival, the nurse ensures that the procedure is understood by the patient and informed written consent obtained by the referring clinician. Underwear below the waist should be removed and the patient given protective hospital clothing. Bowel preparation is administered as prescribed.

When the bowel is considered satisfactorily prepared, the examination can be carried out. The patient is positioned comfortably in the left lateral position and the drugs of choice administered. The endoscopist should perform digital examination of the rectum before inserting the instrument. During the procedure, the patient is reassured and maintained in the correct position. Any biopsy specimens obtained during the procedure should be handled as previously described. Diathermy may be used to obtain large specimens for histology or to perform polypectomy.

After the examination, the patient is made clean and comfortable and allowed to recover from the effect of the drugs. The equipment is cleaned and disinfected.

Colonoscopy

Check list

Colonoscope and accessories
Light source
Trolley
Suction pump
Gauze swabs
Lubricant
Disposable gloves
Drugs: diazepam ⎤
      pethidine ⎬ for intravenous administration if required
      naloxone |
      hyoscine (Buscopan) ⎦
Needles
Syringes
Intravenous cannulae
Resuscitation equipment

continued

Diathermy equipment: supply unit
                       snares
                       'hot' biopsy forceps
Arrange radiology screening if this is required by the endoscopist
Check the 10-day rule if appropriate
Histology specimen containers and request forms

Procedure

The patient may be an inpatient or outpatient depending on the clinical state and the method of bowel preparation prescribed. On arrival, the nurse ensures that the procedure is understood by the patient and informed written consent obtained by the referring clinician. Bowel preparation should be carried out

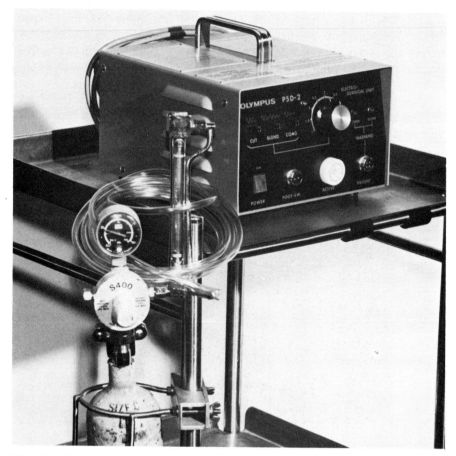

Fig. 7.8 *Diathermy unit with carbon dioxide cylinder, flow meter and tubing in position for use with mannitol bowel preparation.*

until it is considered satisfactory to proceed to colonoscopy. The patient is dressed in a hospital protective gown and positioned comfortably in the left lateral position on a couch or trolley with an incontinence pad under the buttocks. Sedation may be administered via an intravenous cannula. After digital examination of the rectum, the colonoscope is inserted.

During the procedure, the patient is reassured and maintained in the correct position. Any biopsy specimens obtained should be handled as previously described.

If colonic polyps are found during the procedure, histology will definitely be

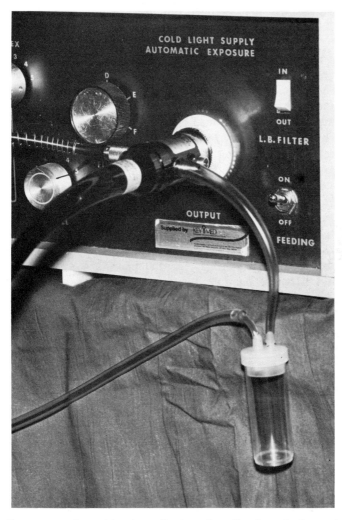

Fig. 7.9 *Sputum trap in position for collection of small polyps via the suction channel of the colonoscope.*

required and if possible the polyps should be excised using diathermy. The equipment should always be available and in good working order for all colonoscopy sessions. Ideally, two nurses should be available during polypectomy. One should look after the patient and one assist the endoscopist. If the polyps removed by diathermy are small, they may be withdrawn from the colon by suction via the colonoscope. In order to retrieve them for histological examination, a sputum trap can be attached to the colonoscope at the suction outlet and then to the suction tubing. This will ensure that small specimens are saved and not lost in the aspirate from the colon (Figs 7.8 and 7.9).

After the procedure, the patient is made clean and comfortable and allowed to rest. If the bowel is very distended with insufflated air, greater comfort may be achieved by allowing the patient to recover in the prone position.

Complications of sigmoidoscopy and colonoscopy

During diagnostic procedures hypotension or respiratory arrest may occur as a result of over-aggressive sedative regimes. Perforation of the colon may occur due to inexperience or the use of excessive force. It may be caused by the tip of the instrument or by a loop formed during the procedure. Diverticula may be perforated by over-inflation. Mucosal haemorrhage is rare during simple diagnostic procedures but mesenteric haemorrhage and rupture of the spleen and liver have been reported secondary to over-vigorous manipulation.

Snare polypectomy is more dangerous than the simple diagnostic procedure. Bleeding from the polyp stalk may be copious, but this complication is rare. Full thickness mural burns may cause perforation, whilst a contralateral burn may cause peritonism and persistent abdominal pain. Rarely, current leakage may cause a burn to the endoscopist, the patient or the assistant. Extra care must be taken in patients who have cardiac pacemakers since the diathermy may interfere with its function. Bacteriaemia has been reported after the procedure but severe septic complications are rare.

8

GASTROINTESTINAL HAEMORRHAGE

ENDOSCOPY IN GASTROINTESTINAL HAEMORRHAGE

Requests for endoscopy in patients who have suffered a gastrointestinal haemorrhage may constitute up to 10% of the work load of an endoscopy unit. There are many problems relating to offering an urgent service to cope with this work load. Patients may be too ill to move, so that endoscopy may need to be performed away from the endoscopy unit, for example on the patient's ward, or even in the operating theatre. A special endoscopy set with endoscope, light source and accessories should always be ready to travel to such a situation, where adequate facilities for cleaning the instrument after endoscopy should also be available. Patients will need to be resuscitated and the blood volume restored before endoscopy. Resuscitation may still be in progress during the endoscopy and care must be taken to ensure that it is maintained and not jeopardized. The presence of fresh blood and blood clot in the stomach may make endoscopy difficult and hazardous. Although gastric lavage need not be contemplated routinely, it may be necessary to evacuate the stomach and wash it out with saline via a large bore stomach tube during the endoscopy.

Colonoscopy may be used to reveal the source of colonic haemorrhage. Emergency colonoscopy is probably under-valued in these circumstances and is less widely practised than it ought to be. Successful localization of the bleeding site, good instrumentation, and a skilled endoscopist are all required. In patients with torrential haemorrhage, no colonic preparation is needed, but other patients will need colonic washouts prior to the procedure. Intraluminal blood and clots adherent to the mucosa will need to be washed away during the procedure to obtain good mucosal views. Proctosigmoidoscopy should be performed prior to colonoscopy to exclude distal lesions and acute colitis which would constitute a contraindication to colonoscopy.

It is usually unnecessary to perform endoscopy immediately the patient is admitted with gastrointestinal haemorrhage. A delay of up to 12 hours often results in cessation of haemorrhage, emptying of clots and blood from the stomach or colon and the success of resuscitative measures. Under normal circumstances, endoscopy should therefore be performed within 24 hours of admission to hospital, when the endoscopy can usually be performed with the regular endoscopy team at hand. Nevertheless, torrential haemorrhage may occasionally require urgent surgery and emergency endoscopy. These endoscopies are the most hazardous and should only be performed by an experienced endoscopist. Some units may be able to establish the facility of an on-call endoscopy assistant to cope with such crises but this is a rarity and much emergency endoscopy is usually supported by non-expert staff from the ward or operating theatre.

The choice of endoscope is important under such circumstances. Since upper gastrointestinal panendoscopy will need to be performed, an end-viewing instrument should be selected. Because copious volumes of gastric contents and fresh blood may need to be aspirated, a large endoscope with a wide suction channel is needed. After the endoscopy has been performed, extra care will be required during cleaning to reduce the risk of blockage of the endoscope channels by foreign material.

Various therapeutic techniques may be contemplated during the endoscopy depending upon the diagnosis established. The presence of oesophageal varices may lead to endoscopic sclerotherapy or the placement of a Sengstaken–Blakemore tube. Laser or diathermic coagulation of the bleeding lesion may be considered, or drugs designed to reduce haemorrhage may be applied to the bleeding mucosa. The endoscopy assistant should be prepared for any of these eventualities.

Nursing care during OGD

(1) Ensure that there are at least two nurses available to assist at the examination

(2) A nurse from the patient's ward would also be helpful to assist with the care of the patient

(3) Adequate suction must be available for the endoscope and for mouth aspiration

(4) It is necessary to provide adequate protection for the patient's clothes and bedding, e.g. incontinence pads

(5) All staff should wear disposable gloves during the examination and when handling contaminated equipment

(6) Prepare the endoscopy room and equipment as for routine endoscopy

(7) Ascertain the endoscopist's drug requirements for this examination as they may differ from routine OGD

(8) Contact the ward to arrange the procedure, at the same time establishing the patient's present condition and any special requirements which may be necessary

(9) On receiving the patient, ensure that consent has been obtained and that the procedure has been understood

(10) Check that any intravenous therapy is functioning satisfactorily. Make sure more blood or i.v. solutions are readily available

(11) Local anaesthesia may be omitted if this could promote nausea and subsequent vomiting

(12) The patient is positioned in the left lateral position and made secure to ensure that no stomach contents are inhaled in the event of vomiting. A variable position trolley or table with a head down facility should be used to assist in maintaining the airway and vital functions of the patient

(13) Sedation is administered by the endoscopist and the patient observed carefully. In the severely ill patient sedation may be omitted to minimize adverse drug effects

(14) During the intubation and inspection, one nurse should be responsible for the care of the patient and one nurse for assisting the endoscopist. In the acutely ill bleeding patient, endoscopy can be both dangerous and unsatisfactory if adequate nursing care is not provided

(15) Any therapeutic procedure which may be required must be provided quickly and efficiently

(16) During the inspection and therapeutic phase of this procedure, the nurse looking after the patient is responsible for reporting any visible changes in condition as the endoscopist will be engrossed with the view down the endoscope

(17) After the examination, the patient is made comfortable and regular observations continued

Extra equipment required for therapeutic procedures

Depending on availability and presumed diagnosis:

Varices injection needles and solutions
Diathermy equipment with accessories
Bipolar diathermy system
Laser

Other necessary equipment:

Tipping trolley or table for patient
Adequate efficient suction for mouth aspiration and the endoscope
Intravenous solutions
Pitressin for injection
Pressure infusor for blood or solutions
Sengstaken—Blakemore tube with the necessary accessories for rapid tamponade if required
Resuscitation equipment
Oxygen supply
Tissues

Disposable gloves
Incontinence pads
Bowl containing water to clear suction catheters

Cleaning endoscopy equipment after use in the bleeding situation

Extra care is required to ensure that all residual blood is removed from the endoscope and accessories. *Always wear gloves!*

Special 'tips'

(1) Always ensure that a foam-controlling agent has been added to all suction bottles during this procedure. Blood tends to froth and it can contaminate filters and tubing in the machine

(2) Change the suction jars when the level of contents is becoming unacceptably high as this will help to prevent damage to the machine and ensure that adequate suction is maintained

(3) On removal of the endoscope from the patient, immediately test the air flow and the water flow

(4) Clean with detergent and rinse with clean water as in routine use

(5) Aspirate hydrogen peroxide 10 vols through the suction channel

(6) Remove biopsy valve and set aside for dismantling and cleaning

(7) Pass cleaning brush through suction channel, clean tip of brush before withdrawal. This procedure may be required to be repeated several times

(8) Clean tip of endoscope with soft toothbrush, paying particular attention to any forceps raiser

(9) Attach wash tube and repeat aspiration of hydrogen peroxide through the suction channel, attach syringe and leave channel full

(10) Inject hydrogen peroxide through the air channel (see 'Blocked channels', p. 35)

(11) Half fill water bottle with hydrogen peroxide and depress water button to ensure good flow through the water channel

(12) Leave endoscope with all channels filled with hydrogen peroxide for 20 minutes

(13) Rinse and disinfect as for routine use

Cleaning of accessories

(1) Dismantle as far as possible

(2) Clean with detergent, using a brush for channels and crevices if possible

(3) Soak in hydrogen peroxide 10 vols until all signs of denaturing of protein matter have stopped

(4) An ultrasonic machine is very helpful in agitating out all residual debris

(5) Rinse and disinfect as for routine use

Insertion of a Sengstaken–Blakemore tube

Check list

Sengstaken tube − with correct connections and in good working order (Fig. 8.1)
Artery forceps − 4 pairs
Gauze swabs
Lubricant
30 ml syringe − to fill balloons
Water ⎤
Contrast medium ⎬ to fill balloons
Sphygmomanometer ⎦
Suction equipment for mouth aspiration
Tissues
Non-sterile drapes or incontinence pads
Disposable gloves

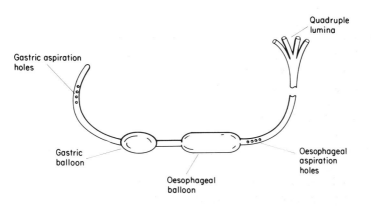

Fig. 8.1 *Modified Sengstaken–Blakemore tube, showing quadruple tubing for aspiration from stomach and oesophagus, and inflation of gastric and oesophageal balloons.*

Procedure

The doctor should test both the oesophageal and gastric balloons prior to insertion of the tube and confirm patency of the gastric aspiration channel.

With the patient positioned in the left lateral position, a local anaesthetic spray is applied to the hypopharynx. The previously lubricated Sengstaken tube should then be passed through the hypopharynx and into the oesophagus. Advancement is continued until the gastric balloon is well into the body of the stomach as indicated by distance markings on the external wall of the tube.

During this phase of the procedure mouth aspiration may have to be undertaken to minimize retention of regurgitated secretions.

With the gastric balloon well positioned in the body of the stomach, it should be inflated with 100 ml of water and 30 ml of radio-opaque contrast medium. The Sengstaken tube should then be pulled back at the mouth until resistance to further withdrawal is experienced. At this stage, the gastric balloon fits snuggly in the fundus of the stomach. The oesophageal balloon should now be inflated with air to a pressure of 35–40 mm Hg. This pressure may be checked using a sphygmomanometer. Both gastric and oesophageal inflation tubes should be occluded with two pairs of artery forceps. Once this has been performed the Sengstaken tube should be firmly tethered to the face. An additional refinement is to place a fine oesophageal tube with its lumen proximal to the inflated oesophageal balloon. Through it, continuous oesophageal aspiration may be undertaken. The gastric contents may be aspirated via the aspiration channel of the Sengstaken tube.

After the procedure, light sedation may need to be given to the patient since the tube produces considerable discomfort.

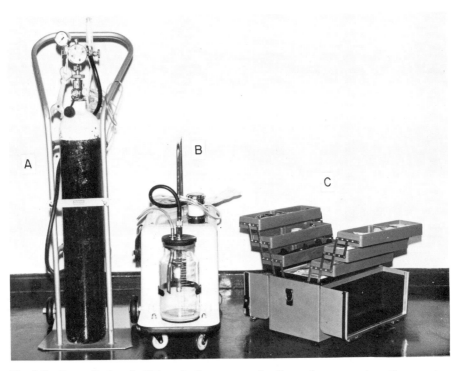

Fig. 8.2   Resuscitation facilities. A, Oxygen supply; B, suction apparatus; C, resuscitation box containing resuscitation equipment and drugs.

RESUSCITATION PROCEDURE IN THE GASTROENTEROLOGY DEPARTMENT

All Gastroenterology departments require an adequate supply of resuscitation equipment to comply with hospital resuscitation policy (Fig. 8.2)
The department staff must be familiar with:

The equipment in the department
The routine resuscitation procedure
The telephone number for the cardiac arrest team

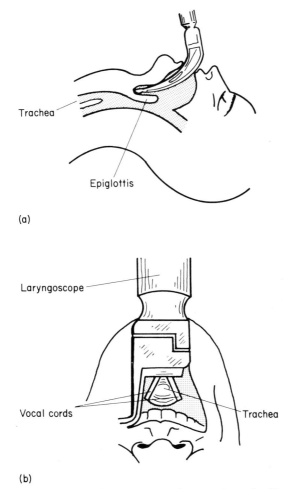

(a)

(b)

Fig. 8.3 *(a) Correct position of laryngoscope prior to endotracheal intubation. (b) View of trachea and vocal cords which should be obtained prior to endotracheal intubation.*

Cardiac and respiratory arrests may occur in the Gastroenterology department as in any other hospital area. Particular problems which may be precipitated by drug administration or invasive procedure in the Gastroenterology department are:

(1) *Respiratory arrest:* as a reaction to intravenous diazepam
(2) *Cardiac arrhythmias:* as a reaction to atropine or diazepam
(3) *Vomiting:* (a) in cases of pyloric stenosis
          (b) in cases of gastrointestinal haemorrhage
(4) *Collapse:* (a) as a vasovagal reaction to the prospect of an invasive procedure
         (b) as a result of gastrointestinal haemorrhage

These problems require routine care as for the unconscious patient and immediate medical attention. The nurse in charge of the department is responsible for:

(1) Ensuring that the resuscitation equipment is available, complete and in good working order
(2) Ensuring that there is correctly functioning suction equipment and oxygen supply in the department
(3) Ensuring that all staff are familiar with the resuscitation procedure and have attended in-service training in this subject (Figs 8.3 and 8.4).

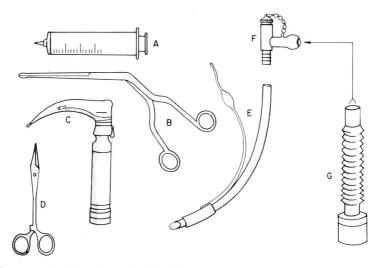

Fig. 8.4 *Apparatus for endotracheal intubation. A, 20 ml syringe; B, Magill intubating forceps; C, Macintosh laryngoscope; D, Spencer-Wells artery forceps; E, cuffed endotracheal tube; F, Cobb's connector; G, corrugated catheter mount.*

Adult resuscitation equipment

 1. Laryngoscope
 2. Plastic laryngoscope
 3. 2 spare batteries
 4. 2 spare bulbs
 5. Cuffed endo-tracheal tubes 7.0; 8.0; 9.0: 2 of each
 6. 2 corrugated catheter mounts
 7. Introducing forceps
 8. Adjustable metal introducer
 9. Silastic introducer
10. Artery forceps
11. 20 ml syringe with adaptor
12. Endo-tracheal tube lubrication
13. Airways sizes 2, 3 and 4
14. Mouth gag
15. Face masks sizes 4, 5 and 6
16. 2 angle pieces for oxygen tubing
17. Non-return valve with oxygen attachment and re-breathing bag
18. Ambu-bag
19. Suction probes
20. Endo-bronchial suction catheters
21. Assorted intravenous cannulae, needles and syringes
22. Sodium bicarbonate 8.4% and giving set
23. Adhesive strapping and scissors
24. Drugs supplied by pharmacy
25. Green oxygen connecting tubing
26. Intravenous infusion set
27. 500 ml dextrose 5%
28. Brook airway

BIBLIOGRAPHY AND USEFUL ADDRESSES

Book list

Bennett, J. R. (ed.) (1981) *Therapeutic Endoscopy and Radiology of the Gut*, Chapman and Hall, London.

Cotton, P. B. and Williams, C. B. (1982) *Practical Gastrointestinal Endoscopy*, Blackwell's Scientific Publications, Oxford.

Drossman, D. A. (1982) *Manual of Gastroenterological Procedures*, Raven Press, New York.

Hollanders, D. (1979) *Gastrointestinal Endoscopy: An Introduction for Assistants*, Bailliere Tindall, London.

Hunt, R. H. and Waye, J. D. (eds) (1981) *Colonoscopy: Techniques, Clinical Practice and Colour Atlas*, Chapman and Hall, London and Year Book, Chicago.

Salmon, P. R. (1974) *Fibre-Optic Endoscopy*, Pitman Medical, London.

Schiller, K. F. R. and Salmon, P. R. (eds) (1976) *Modern Topics in Gastrointestinal Fibre-Endoscopy*, William Heinemann Medical, London.

Swan, C. H. J. (ed.) (1981) *A Handbook of Gastrointestinal Endoscopy*, Endoscopy Committee of the British Society of Gastroenterology, London.

Useful addresses

Endoscopy Assistants Group
Secretariat, British Society of Gastroenterology
Rayne Institute
University College Hospital
5 University Street
London WC1

Association of Nursing Practice
Royal College of Nursing
Henrietta Place
London

Society of Gastrointestinal Assistants
211E 43rd Street
New York
NY 10017
USA

European Society of Gastrointestinal Endoscopy
Zuchwilerstrasse 43
4500 Solothurn
Switzerland

Organisation Mondiale D'Endoscopie Digestive
c/o The First Department of Internal Medicine
Faculty of Medicine
University of Tokyo 3/1
7 Chome
Hongo
Bunkyo-Ku
Tokyo 113
Japan

APPENDIX A
ENDOSCOPY AND INFECTION

This is a reprint of the 'Report and Recommendations of the Endoscopy Committee of the British Society of Gastroenterology, accepted by the Annual Business Meeting of Members, Exeter, September 1981.'

There are numerous published and unpublished reports of serious infection related to gastrointestinal endoscopy. The Endoscopy Committee is increasingly concerned about the lack of awareness of this problem. In 1980, a survey of 52 large endoscopy units showed that less than half were using effective disinfecting schedules. These recommendations are based on a detailed review of the literature, workshops involving endoscopists, microbiologists, instrument and disinfection experts, and on comments received following discussion of a draft document circulated in April 1981.

Microbiological hazards during endoscopy

(1) Patient to patient transfer

Organisms can be carried from patient to patient on contaminated endoscopes. There have been several *Salmonella* epidemics. Opportunistic organisms such as *Pseudomonas* frequently colonize endoscopic equipment which has not been adequately disinfected, and such organisms have been instilled into a succession of patients during endoscopy lists. This passage has resulted in serious primary infections in patients whose immunity is compromised and during routine ERCP when contaminated contrast is injected into stagnant duct systems. A similar mechanism could lead to intestinal colonization, with resulting spread of antibiotic resistant organisms throughout a hospital. There is a theoretical hazard of transmitting virus infections such as hepatitis, but no reported cases.

(2) Bacteraemia

Gastrointestinal endoscopy (like many other investigative procedures) can result in transient bacteraemia; there is a theoretical risk of endocarditis in susceptible individuals.

(3) Aspiration pneumonia

Regurgitation and inhalation of stomach contents may result in pneumonia and lung abscess.

(4) Risks to staff of endoscopy units

These risks include overt infections from contact with blood, sputum and gastrointestinal fluids, and the potential hazard of acquiring antibiotic resistant flora.

Methods for disinfecting endoscopes

(1) Fibrescopes cannot be formally sterilized.

(2) Assiduous cleaning is more important than the use of specific disinfectants. Instruments are complex and effective cleaning requires staff with appropriate training, time and motivation. Instrument manufacturers and their agents make appropriate recommendations. The process may be facilitated in the future by semi-automatic washing and disinfection machines.

(3) Disinfectants. So far, only gluteraldehyde and povidone-iodine have been shown to provide effective disinfection in endoscopy units. Unfortunately, skin sensitivity to gluteraldehyde appears to be a common problem in British endoscopy units and povidone-iodine is unpleasant to use and may stain the equipment. 70% alcohol has been recommended as an alternative and does have proven activity when used after obsessional cleaning. 70% alcohol may damage the bending section of the endoscope when used externally and can constitute a fire hazard. Experiments are being conducted with hypochlorite solutions and various quaternary ammonium compounds.

Recommendations

(1) Equipment

(a) Endoscopy should be performed only with properly cleaned and disinfected equipment.

(b) Definition and validation of disinfection methods. The methods used in a particular unit should be laid down in collaboration with the hospital microbiologist and infection control officer with reference to the published literature and manufacturer's instructions. The effectiveness of the chosen cleaning and disinfection procedures should be checked by regular microbiological surveys. A method of proven value is outlined below.

(c) Instruments are cleaned according to the manufacturer's instructions. The instrument shaft, suction channel, air channel and water channel are then soaked in an effective disinfectant for at least 10 minutes. Ancillary equipment is equally important. All ancillaries are dismantled as far as possible and cleaned with a brush and detergent. An ultrasonic cleaning tank is useful. Sterilization is aimed for wherever possible. The following equipment can be autoclaved: biopsy valves, ERCP catheters (but not stilettes), cytology brushes, metal dilators, splinting tubes, cleaning brushes, bowls, receivers etc. The following cannot withstand autoclaving and should be disinfected by low temperature steam or immersed in a suitable disinfectant (e.g. gluteraldehyde) for as long as possible: sphincterotomy knives, biopsy forceps, toothguards, water bottles, stiffening tubes, catheter stilettes. Equipment can become significantly contaminated during storage especially if any water is left in the channels. These procedures are therefore followed before as well as after endoscopy lists. Except during lists of potentially infected patients (e.g. sphincterotomy for gallstones), the disinfection procedure between endoscopies is often quicker − provided that the regime is bacteriologically validated. Between cases the instrument is cleaned with a detergent; the suction channel is brushed through; the tip of the instrument is cleaned with a toothbrush; the air/water channel is flushed with water and then air; the shaft of the instrument is immersed in an effective disinfectant which is aspirated into the suction channel and left for 2 minutes before being rinsed with water and dried. A fresh disinfected biopsy valve is used for each examination.

(d) Infected patients. An instrument which has been used in a patient with a communicable disease e.g. salmonellosis, hepatitis, giardiasis, tuberculosis requires special attention. It should be cleaned in the usual way and then exposed thoroughly to disinfectant (e.g. gluteraldehyde) for at least 2 hours. Alternatively, it can be sterilized using ethylene oxide gas at low pressure after vigorous cleaning.

(2) Staff and facilities

(a) All endoscopists and endoscopy assistants should be made fully aware of the dangers of using contaminated instruments and should be trained specifically in the care, cleaning and sterilization of endoscopic equipment.

(b) Certain minimum standards for endoscopy rooms should be established, bearing in mind the health and safety of staff as well as patients.

(c) Staff should be aware of the dangers of sensitivity to disinfectants. Suitable precautions must be made to avoid splashing and staff should wear gloves when exposed.

(3) Patients

(a) Immunosuppressed patients. Patients who are effectively immunosuppressed are at a greater risk of infective complications. The indication for endoscopy should be reviewed critically: special care should be exercised with a disinfection technique and the use of prophylactic antibiotics considered.

(b) Endocarditis. There is a theoretical danger of endocarditis developing following gastrointestinal instrumentation in patients with valvular heart disease and antibiotic prophylaxis has been suggested by analogy with dental procedures. Review of the literature indicated that there are great difficulties in defining real risks and relevant policies and the committee finds no evidence to support a recommendation for routine antibiotic prophylaxis at present.

(c) ERCP. The use of inadequately disinfected equipment carries particular infection risks in patients submitted to ERCP, especially those with stagnant duct systems (e.g. pancreatic cysts, benign or malignant biliary and pancreatic duct stenosis). The introduction of organisms such as *Pseudomonas* has led to severe septic complications and death. The importance of careful disinfection procedures in these cases cannot be overemphasized. Many patients with duct stones have bile infected with enteric organisms. Most endoscopists recommend prophylactic antibiotics (e.g. gentamycin, and ampicillin) when stagnant ducts or cysts are apparent before or at ERCP: some do not use antibiotics for routine sphincterotomy if the duct is cleared.

(4) Research

Further studies are necessary on many aspects of this problem e.g. simplification of instruments to facilitate cleaning and disinfection; better disinfectant solutions and machines; prophylactic antibiotics; protection for staff; certification of endoscopy assistants.

Implications of the recommendations

Those units which have not (yet) experienced infective problems may question the need for these recommendations and consider them to be impractical in a busy environment. Many infectious outbreaks have not been officially reported, but there are sufficient publications to indicate that endoscopy with contaminated equipment can be disastrous. There are major medico-legal implications. The Endoscopy Committee considers that a new emphasis is necessary. It is no longer adequate to do only what local circumstances permit, but essential to press for the resources to make practicable that which is necessary. This may well mean the appointment of more endoscopy nursing staff, alterations to endoscopy areas and the purchase of more instruments and accessories.

APPENDIX B
PATIENT INFORMATION AND
DOCUMENTATION

Appointment forms

It is important that patients attending for gastroenterological investigations should be given adequate information about the procedure to ensure correct physical and psychological preparation.

The referring clinician is responsible for explaining verbally the reasons for any tests or therapeutic procedure necessary for the patient. Written instructions may then be given to the patient to take away to read or sent by mail if that is appropriate.

Any written instructions should be simple to understand and contain relevant information such as date and time of appointment, location of the department and a brief explanation of the procedure and any likely after-effects.

The nurse receiving the patient must ascertain that the information has been understood and that any instructions given have been complied with.

The following are examples of appointment letters which are used for investigations and procedures described in the book.

North Staffordshire Health Authority

CITY GENERAL HOSPITAL

NEWCASTLE ROAD
STOKE-ON-TRENT
ST4 6QG

Enquiries to :

....

Your Ref.
Our Ref.

Telephone
Newcastle, Staffs 621133

Ext. 2214/2265

Department of Gastroenterology

Dear...

Appointment for Gastrointestinal Endoscopy

Arrangements have been made for you to have an endoscopic examination of your stomach on............................ ...., the... 19 ... .,

at .... a.m./p.m. in the Department of Gastroenterology, Ward 71, City General Hospital.

YOU SHOULD HAVE NOTHING TO EAT OR DRINK FOR EIGHT HOURS PRIOR TO YOUR EXAMINATION.

The examination is simple and takes about thirty minutes. You will be given an injection to make your mouth dry, a local anaesthetic spray to your throat and an injection in your arm to make you drowsy. You should be able to return home in approximately 2 hours.

After the examination you will be sleepy for a short time and it is important that you make satisfactory arrangements for your transport home as the effect of the drug may last up to 24-36 hours.

YOU ARE ADVISED NOT TO GO TO WORK, DRIVE A VEHICLE, USE MACHINERY OR DRINK ALCOHOL FOR A FULL DAY FOLLOWING THE EXAMINATION.

If you have any questions or problems related to this appointment, please do not hesitate to contact me on the above telephone number.

Yours sincerely,

Sister
Department of Gastroenterology

Oesophagogastroduodenoscopy

North Staffordshire Health Authority

CITY GENERAL HOSPITAL

NEWCASTLE ROAD
STOKE-ON-TRENT
ST4 6QG

Telephone
Newcastle, Staffs 621133

Ext. 2214/2265

Enquiries to :

....

Your Ref.
Our Ref.

Department of Gastroenterology

Dear...

Appointment for Oesophagoscopy and Dilatation

Arrangements have been made for you to have an examination of your oesophagus (gullet) and dilatation if the doctor finds this is necessary during the examination on...................................... the.. 19 ....,

at........................a.m./p.m. in the Department of Gastroenterology, Ward 71, City General Hospital.

YOU SHOULD HAVE NOTHING TO EAT OR DRINK FOR EIGHT HOURS PRIOR TO YOUR EXAMINATION.

The examination is simple and takes about thirty minutes. You will be given an injection to make your mouth dry, a local anaesthetic spray to your throat and an injection in your arm to make you drowsy. You should be able to return home in approximately 3 hours.

After the examination you will be sleepy for a short time and it is important that you make satisfactory arrangements for your transport home as the effect of the drug may last up to 24-36 hours.

YOU ARE ADVISED NOT TO GO TO WORK, DRIVE A VEHICLE, USE MACHINERY OR DRINK ALCOHOL FOR A FULL DAY FOLLOWING THE EXAMINATION.

If you have any questions or problems related to this appointment, please do not hesitate to contact me on the above telephone number.

Yours sincerely,

Sister
Department of Gastroenterology

Oesophagoscopy/Dilatation

North Staffordshire Health Authority

CITY GENERAL HOSPITAL

NEWCASTLE ROAD
STOKE-ON-TRENT
ST4 6QG

Enquiries to :

....

Your Ref.
Our Ref.

Telephone
Newcastle. Staffs 621133

Ext. 2214/2265

Department of Gastroenterology

Dear...

Appointment for Oesophagoscopy and Insertion of Oesophageal Tube

Arrangements have been made for you to have an endoscopic examination of your oesophagus (gullet) and insertion of a tube if the doctor finds this necessary on .... at..........................
in the Department of Gastroenterology, Ward 71, City General Hospital.

YOU SHOULD HAVE NOTHING TO EAT OR DRINK FOR EIGHT HOURS PRIOR TO YOUR EXAMINATION.

The examination is simple and takes about thirty minutes. You will be given an injection to make your mouth dry, a local anaesthetic spray to your throat and an injection in your arm to make you drowsy. You should be able to return home in approximately 2 hours.

After the examination you will be sleepy for a short time and it is important that you make satisfactory arrangements for your transport home as the effect of the drug may last up to 24-36 hours. You may be kept in hospital overnight after this procedure so please come prepared for this.

YOU ARE ADVISED NOT TO GO TO WORK, DRIVE A VEHICLE, USE MACHINERY OR DRINK ALCOHOL FOR A FULL DAY FOLLOWING THE EXAMINATION.

If you have any questions or problems related to this appointment. please do not hesitate to contact me on the above telephone number.

Yours sincerely.

Sister
Department of Gastroenterology

Oesophagoscopy/Intubation

North Staffordshire Health Authority
CITY GENERAL HOSPITAL
NEWCASTLE ROAD
STOKE-ON-TRENT
ST4 6QG

Telephone
Newcastle, Staffs 621133

Ext. 2214/2265

Enquiries to :

....

Your Ref.
Our Ref.

Department of Gastroenterology

Dear..

Appointment for Gastrointestinal Endoscopy with X-rays

Arrangements have been made for you to have an examination of your stomach, the first part of your bowel and your biliary and pancreatic ducts on

.... the .... at .... a.m./p.m. in the Department of Gastroenterology, Ward 7, City General Hospital.

YOU SHOULD HAVE NOTHING TO EAT OR DRINK FOR EIGHT HOURS PRIOR TO YOUR EXAMINATION.

You will be given an injection to make your mouth dry, a local anaesthetic spray to your throat and and injection in your arm to make you drowsy. The doctor will then ask you to swallow a flexible tube through which he can see to carry out the examination.

During the procedure you will be X-rayed. If you are female and of child-bearing age, please ensure you are within the first 10 days of your menstrual cycle and not pregnant as X-rays may be a hazard in pregnancy. Please also let us know if you have a cardiac pacemaker fitted, as we may use diathermy current during the procedure and this could interfere with the pacemaker.

After the examination you will be sleepy for a short time. You may be able to return home on the same day or may need to be kept in hospital overnight. Please ensure you make satisfactory arrangements for your transport home. The effect of the drugs used last 24-36 hours.

YOU ARE ADVISED NOT TO GO TO WORK, DRIVE A VEHICLE, USE MACHINERY OR DRINK ALCOHOL FOR A FULL DAY FOLLOWING THE EXAMINATION.

If you have any questions or problems related to this appointment please do not hesitate to contact me on the above telephone number.

Yours sincerely,

Sister
Department of Gastroenterology

E.R.C.P./
Sphincterotomy

North Staffordshire Health Authority
CITY GENERAL HOSPITAL
NEWCASTLE ROAD
STOKE-ON-TRENT
ST4 6QG

Enquiries to :

....

Your Ref.
Our Ref.

Telephone
Newcastle, Staffs 621133

Ext. 2214/2265

Department of Gastroenterology

Dear...

Arrangements have been made for you to have an examination of your bowel on.., in the Department of Gastroenterology.

You may be able to return home on the same day at approximately 4-00 p.m., or you may need to be kept in hospital overnight.

The test involves the passage of a flexible tube into the back passage and normally takes about thirty minutes.

In order to ensure your bowel is clean before the examination, you are asked to :

1. Observe the diet restrictions on the enclosed sheet.

2. Take the four enclosed (Senokot) tablets as instructed on the enclosed sheet.

3. Be prepared to arrive at 9.00 a.m. on the date above and spend the morning in the Gastroenterology Department, drinking a special purgative fluid followed by further quantities of clear fluid until the bowel is clear.

To make you comfortable during the examination you will be given a sedative injection. The effect of this drug may last 24-36 hours. Therefore you are advised not to drink alcohol, drive a motor vehicle or work with machinery during that period.

You should make satisfactory arrangements for your transport home after the examination.

If you have any queries do not hesitate to telephone me on the above number.

Yours sincerely,

Sister
Department of Gastroenterology

COLONOSCOPY (1)

North Staffordshire Health Authority

CITY GENERAL HOSPITAL
NEWCASTLE ROAD
STOKE-ON-TRENT
ST4 6QG

Enquiries to:

....

Your Ref.

Our Ref.

Telephone
Newcastle, Staffs 621133

Ext ....

Department of Gastroenterology

Dear...................................,

It has been arranged for you to have an examination of your bowel
on .... 19.... Please come to the Department
of Gastroenterology (Ward 71) at the City General Hospital at ....

In order to ensure that your bowel is empty and prepared for the
inspection please follow this regime:

48 hours before the day of the examination i.e. after .... on
...................................., take only a fluid diet.

Between 2.00 p.m. and 4.00 p.m. on the day before the examination,
please take the "X-Prep" liquid which is with this letter.

After 10.00 p.m. on the evening before the examination please drink
only water, but do not take any fluids on the morning of the examination.

On arrival in the department you will be given an enema to ensure your
bowel is empty.

Before the examination you will be given an injection to make you drowsy.
Because of this, you should arrange for someone to drive you home and you
are advised to:

AVOID ALCOHOL, WORKING WITH MACHINERY AND DRIVING FOR AT LEAST 24 HOURS
AFTER THE EXAMINATION.

If this appointment is inconvenient or you have any further queries
please do not hesitate to telephone me on the above number.

Yours sincerely,

Sister
Department of Gastroenterology

Colonoscopy (2)

North Staffordshire Health Authority

CITY GENERAL HOSPITAL

Enquiries to :

....

Your Ref.

Our Ref.

NEWCASTLE ROAD
STOKE-ON-TRENT
ST4 6QG

Telephone
Newcastle, Staffs 621133

Ext. 2214/2265

Department of Gastroenterology

Dear...

Arrangements have been made for you to have an examination of your bowel on

.... at..............................in the Department of Gastroenterology (Ward 71) at the City General Hospital. You should be able to return home on the same day.

The test involves the passage of a flexible tube into the back passage and normally takes about thirty minutes. On arrival for the examination you will be given an enema to ensure the bowel is clean before the examination.

Two suppositories are enclosed along with instructions so that you may use them correctly. Please use them the night before the examination.

It is *possible* you may have a sedative injection before the examination; it is therefore advisable for you to make satisfactory arrangements for your transport home, usually after 1—2 hours. The effect of the drug used lasts 24—36 hours, so YOU ARE ADVISED NOT TO GO TO WORK, DRIVE A VEHICLE, USE MACHINERY OR DRINK ALCOHOL FOR A FULL DAY FOLLOWING THE EXAMINATION.

If you have any questions or problems related to this appointment, please do not hesitate to contact me on the above telephone numbers.

Yours sincerely,

Sister
Department of Gastroenterology

Fibresigmoidoscopy

North Staffordshire Health Authority
CITY GENERAL HOSPITAL
NEWCASTLE ROAD
STOKE-ON-TRENT
ST4 6QG

Enquiries to :

Telephone
Newcastle, Staffs 621133

Ext. 2214/2265

Your Ref.
Our Ref.

Department of Gastroenterology

Dear..

Arrangements have been made for you to have an examination of your bowel on .... at...................a.m./p.m. in the Department of Gastroenterology, Ward 71, City General Hospital.

This involves the passage of a small telescope into the back passage and normally takes about ten minutes.

Please eat only a light breakfast if you are coming in the morning or a light lunch if your appointment is in the afternoon.

Two suppositories are enclosed along with instructions so that you may use them correctly and ensure your bowel is empty for the examination.

If you have any questions or problems related to this appointment, please do not hesitate to contact me on the above telephone number.

Yours sincerely.

Sister
Department of Gastroenterology

Rigid Sigmoidoscopy

North Staffordshire Health Authority
CITY GENERAL HOSPITAL
NEWCASTLE ROAD
STOKE-ON-TRENT
ST4 6QG

Enquiries to :

Telephone
Newcastle, Staffs 621133

Ext. 2214/2265

Your Ref.
Our Ref.

Department of Gastroenterology

Dear...

Arrangements have been made for you to have a special test on your bowel

performed on .... at............................. in the
Department of Gastroenterology (Ward 71) at the City General Hospital.

This involves the swallowing of a thin tube with a small capsule on the end,
followed by X-rays to determine its position before a specimen is taken. If you are
female and of child-bearing age, please ensure you are within the first 10 days of
your menstrual cycle and not pregnant, as X-rays can be a hazard in pregnancy.

YOU MUST NOT EAT OR DRINK ANYTHING FOR EIGHT HOURS BEFORE
THE TEST.

If you have any questions or problems related to this appointment, please do not
hesitate to contact me on the above telephone numbers.

Yours sincerely,

Sister
Department of Gastroenterology

Jejunal Biopsy

North Staffordshire Health Authority
CITY GENERAL HOSPITAL
NEWCASTLE ROAD
STOKE-ON-TRENT
ST4 6QG

Telephone
Newcastle, Staffs 621133

Ext. 2214/2265

Enquiries to :

....

Your Ref.
Our Ref.

Department of Gastroenterology

Dear..

Arrangements have been made for you to have a...

test on.. at...........................
in the Department of Gastroenterology (Ward 71) at the City General Hospital.

This requires a tube being passed into your stomach through your nose or
mouth followed by the collection of specimens from the tube, and normally lasts a
couple of hours. In order to make sure the tube is in the correct position, you may
be X-rayed. If you are female and of child-bearing age, please ensure you are within
the first 10 days of your menstrual cycle and not pregnant, as X-rays can be a
hazard in pregnancy. You will be given an injection and a liquid meal as part of
the test.

YOU MUST NOT EAT OR DRINK ANYTHING FOR EIGHT HOURS BEFORE
THE TEST.

You will be in the hospital most of the morning. If you have any questions or
problems related to this appointment, please do not hesitate to contact me on the
above telephone number.

Yours sincerely,

Sister
Department of Gastroenterology

Pancreatic function test
Hollander test
Pentagastrin test

North Staffordshire Health Authority

CITY GENERAL HOSPITAL

NEWCASTLE ROAD
STOKE-ON-TRENT
ST4 6QG

Enquiries to :

Telephone
Newcastle, Staffs 621133

Ext. 2214/2265

Your Ref.
Our Ref.

Department of Gastroenterology

Dear..

Arrangements have been made for you to have a pancreatic function test on

.... at................................

This does not require swallowing a tube. You will be given a milk drink as part of the test and asked to collect all urine passed for the next 6 hours. It is important that you do not take any of the following substances for 24 hours prior to the test:

Prunes

Cranberries

Anchovies

Diuretics (water tablets)

Sulphonamides (urinary antibiotics)

Paracetomal (Panadol)

Alcohol

YOU MUST NOT EAT OR DRINK ANYTHING FROM 9-00 p.m. THE NIGHT BEFORE THE TEST.

If you are unable to attend, please telephone the above number immediately.

Yours sincerely,

Sister
Department of Gastroenterology

Para–Amino–Benzoic Acid Test

North Staffordshire Health Authority

CITY GENERAL HOSPITAL

NEWCASTLE ROAD
STOKE-ON-TRENT
ST4 6QG

Telephone
Newcastle, Staffs 621133

Ext. 2214/2265

Department of Gastroenterology

Dear...

Arrangements have been made for you to have a breath test in the above

Department on ....

at ....

The test involves swallowing a special mixture followed by a small meal. You will then be asked to sit quietly for four hours and several short collections of your breath made. It should be finished in 4-5 hours.

YOU MUST NOT EAT OR DRINK ANYTHING FOR EIGHT HOURS BEFORE THE TEST.

Please bring something to read.

If you have any questions or problems related to this appointment, please do not hesitate to contact me on the above telephone number.

Yours sincerely,

Sister
Department of Gastroenterology

Breath test

Additional information for patients

It may be necessary to include some additional information for special reasons. For example, the warning about a cardiac pacemaker and diathermy current and the 10-day rule warning could apply for colonoscopy patients and it may be requested by the clinician that medication be stopped for a period of time prior to gastric function tests. Examples of these instructions are shown.

North Staffordshire Health Authority

CITY GENERAL HOSPITAL

NEWCASTLE ROAD
STOKE-ON-TRENT
ST4 6QG

Telephone
Newcastle, Staffs 621133

Enquiries to :

Ext......................

Your Ref.
Our Ref.

Please do not take any antacid tablets or ulcer healing drugs

for 24 hours prior to attending for this test.

North Staffordshire Health Authority

CITY GENERAL HOSPITAL

NEWCASTLE ROAD
STOKE-ON-TRENT
ST4 6QG

Enquiries to :

Telephone
Newcastle. Staffs 62113ა

Ext

Your Ref.

Our Ref.

You may be subjected to X-rays during this procedure. If you are female and of child-bearing age, please ensure you are within the first 10 days of your menstrual cycle and not pregnant. as X-rays can be a hazard in pregnancy.

or

North Staffordshire Health Authority

CITY GENERAL HOSPITAL

NEWCASTLE ROAD
STOKE-ON-TRENT
ST4 6QG

Enquiries to :

Telephone
Newcastle. Staffs 62113.

Ext

Your Ref.

Our Ref.

Please let us know if you have a cardiac pacemaker fitted as diathermy current could interfere with the pacemaker.

Information for the patient to take home

During a large number of gastrointestinal investigations and procedures, patients will be sedated with diazepam. This may cause amnesia in some patients which will mean that any information given verbally after the procedure may be forgotten. It is useful to give a brief information sheet to the patient prior to discharge home. This can be subsequently referred to by the patient and relatives. Examples of these information sheets are shown here.

North Staffordshire Health Authority

CITY GENERAL HOSPITAL

NEWCASTLE ROAD
STOKE-ON-TRENT
ST4 6QG

Telephone
Newcastle, Staffs 621133

Ext. 2214/2265

Enquiries to :

....

Your Ref.
Our Ref.

Department of Gastroenterology

O.G.D./E.R.C.P.

Today, you have had a gastrointestinal endoscopy. You are unlikely to have any serious after-effects but :

1. If you have a sore throat, this should be only slight and pass off quickly.

2. If you have any discomfort in your arm into which the sedative injection was given, please let me know.

3. If you have any abdominal discomfort this is most likely due to the air the doctor put in during the examination and this effect will not last long.

Should you be worried about these or any other problems related to the examination, please do not hesitate to get in touch. If it is after 5.00 p.m. you are advised to contact your own doctor.

REMEMBER THE WARNING GIVEN TO YOU ON YOUR APPOINTMENT LETTER REGARDING THE SEDATIVE INJECTION.

Your General Practitioner will receive a report regarding the examination within 10 days.

North Staffordshire Health Authority

CITY GENERAL HOSPITAL

NEWCASTLE ROAD
STOKE-ON-TRENT
ST4 6QG

Enquiries to :

....

Your Ref.

Our Ref.

Telephone
Newcastle, Staffs 621133

Ext. 2214/2265

Department of Gastroenterology

OESOPHAGOSCOPY AND DILATATION

Today, you have had a gastrointestinal endoscopy. You are unlikely to have any serious after-effects but :

1. If you have a sore throat, this should be only slight and pass off quickly.

2. If you have any discomfort in your arm into which the sedative injection was given, please let me know.

3. If you have any discomfort in your chest and upper part of your abdomen, it is most likely due to the stretching of your gullet and this effect will not last long.

SHOULD THE LATTER PROBLEM PERSIST OR INCREASE, PLEASE CONTACT US — IF AFTER 5-00 p.m. YOU SHOULD CONTACT YOUR OWN DOCTOR.

REMEMBER THE WARNING GIVEN TO YOU ON YOUR APPOINTMENT LETTER REGARDING THE SEDATIVE INJECTION.

Your General Practitioner will receive a report regarding the examination within 10 days.

North Staffordshire Health Authority

CITY GENERAL HOSPITAL

NEWCASTLE ROAD

STOKE-ON-TRENT

ST4 6QG

Enquiries to:

....

Your Ref.

Our Ref.

Telephone
Newcastle. Staffs 621133

Ext

Department of Gastroenterology

Advice To Patients Who Have Had An Oesophageal Tube Inserted

Today you have had a tube inserted into your oesophagus (gullet).
This means you will be able to swallow normally and eat most of
the foods you like.

It is advisable that you sleep with your shoulders raised on two
or three pillows to prevent discomfort from stomach acid flowing
back up the tube. Should acid be a problem, do not hesitate to
contact your doctor or this department, as a simple antacid should
help prevent too much discomfort.

In order to make sure the tube does not get blocked we give you
the following advice:

1.   Chew all solid food at least TWICE as long as you
     would do normally.

2.   Sip fizzy drinks during and after each meal.

3.   Make sure you have a reasonable amount of nourishing
     foods each day by liquidising soups, stews and fruit
     if necessary.

If you need any advice about your diet, we can arrange for you
to see the hospital dietitian.

Should you have any trouble with swallowing, please contact this
department on the above telephone number between 8.30 a.m. and
5.00 p.m. Monday to Friday. Outside these hours, please contact
your family practitioner.

North Staffordshire Health Authority

CITY GENERAL HOSPITAL

NEWCASTLE ROAD
STOKE-ON-TRENT
ST4 6QG

Enquiries to :

....

Your Ref.
Our Ref.

Telephone
Newcastle, Staffs 621133

Ext. 2214/2265

Department of Gastroenterology

FIBRESIGMOIDOSCOPY / COLONOSCOPY

Today, you have had an endoscopic examination of your bowel. You are unlikely to have any serious after-effects but :

1. If you have any abdominal discomfort, this is most likely due to the air put in by the doctor during the examination and this effect will not last long.

2. If you have any discomfort in your arm or hand into which the sedative injection was given, please let me know.

3. If you pass small traces of blood from the back passage, this could be because you had "biopsies" taken during the examination. SHOULD THIS PERSIST OR INCREASE, PLEASE CONTACT US. — IF AFTER 5.00 p.m. YOU SHOULD CONTACT YOUR OWN DOCTOR.

Please do not hestitate to get in touch if you are worried about these or any other problems related to the examination.

REMEMBER THE WARNING GIVEN TO YOU ON YOUR APPOINTMENT LETTER REGARDING THE SEDATIVE INJECTION !

Your General Practitioner will receive a report regarding the examination within 10 days.

Home bowel preparation

It may be necessary to give extra information about home bowel preparation. These should be very simple and easily understood and examples of these are shown here.

North Staffordshire Health Authority

CITY GENERAL HOSPITAL

NEWCASTLE ROAD
Enquiries to: STOKE-ON-TRENT
....   ST4 6QG
Your Ref.   Department of Gastroenterology
Our Ref.

Telephone
Newcastle, Staffs 621133

Ext....................

HOW TO USE YOUR SUPPOSITORIES

1. Wash your hands.

2. Remove any paper or foil wrapping or plastic casing from the suppository.

3. Insert the whole suppository gently but firmly into the rectum (back passage) tapered end first. Insert the second suppository in the same way.

4. Wash your hands again.

   Squatting or standing with one leg on a chair and bending forward slightly, may make it easier for you to insert the suppositories.

5. After insertion sit quietly, if possible.

6. Wait at least twenty minutes before emptying the bowels.

   SUPPOSITORIES ARE NOT TO BE TAKEN BY MOUTH.

   KEEP ALL MEDICINES OUT OF THE REACH OF CHILDREN.

   Keep the suppositories in a cool place before use (but not in a refrigerator).

North Staffordshire Health Authority

CITY GENERAL HOSPITAL

NEWCASTLE ROAD

Enquiries to:

STOKE-ON-TRENT

ST4 6QG

Telephone
Newcastle, Staffs 631133
2214
Ext....................

....

Your Ref.

Department of Gastroenterology

Our Ref.

BOWEL PREPARATION INSTRUCTIONS

To ensure that the examination is a success, it is
important that you follow all the instructions set
out below very carefully.

4 days before the examination:

Stop any iron tablets you may be taking, but continue
all other medications and any laxatives you usually
take until you come to hospital.

2 days before the examination:

Eat only light meals of egg, cheese and thin white
bread and butter. Have plenty to drink.

Do not eat meat, fish, fruit or vegetables in any form.

1 day before the examination:

Take the 4 enclosed tablets between 2.00 - 3.00 p.m.

On the morning of the examination you may have a
light breakfast of tea and toast if you wish.

(MANNITOL)

North Staffordshire Health Authority

CITY GENERAL HOSPITAL

NEWCASTLE ROAD
STOKE-ON-TRENT
ST4 6QG

Enquiries to:

....

Your Ref.

Our Ref.

Telephone
Newcastle, Staffs 621133

Ext ....

Department of Gastroenterology

Patient Instructions for Bowel Preparation with Sodium Picosulphate (Picolax):

During the two days before your examination you should have only light meals e.g. eggs, cheese, fish, white bread and butter. You should avoid meat, fruit and vegetables in any form.

On the day before your examination: At 7.30 in the morning, dissolve 1 sachet of powder into half a cup of cold water and leave the mixture for five minutes to cool, as the mixture will become hot. Fill the cup with cold water and drink it. This will produce several bowel actions during the day. For breakfast you may have clear fluids and one boiled egg and a slice of white bread and butter. You may drink clear fluids throughout the day. At 12.00 midday, take a light lunch with no vegetables or potatoes, e.g. eggs, cheese, fish, white bread and butter.

At 2.30 in the afternoon, again dissolve 1 sachet of powder into half a cup of water and leave the mixture for five minutes to cool, and fill the cup up with cold water and drink it. Drink only clear fluids for the rest of the day. On the morning of the examination you can have something to drink, but have nothing at all to eat.

Documentation

Consent for investigations and therapeutic procedures: this may be obtained on a specially designed form or on a routine hospital operation consent form (see page 249). It is important that the hospital policy is adhered to and any consent form completed accurately prior to insertion in the case notes of the patient.

Report of investigations and therapeutic procedures: this may be recorded in various ways. A direct entry in the case notes, a punch-card system, a carbon-copy system (see page 250) or a computer entry may be used. Each method requires accurate completion and careful filing for easy interpretation and retrieval.

Prescription sheet: accurate recording of all medication administered to the patient must be made on both the report form and the prescription sheet (see page 251).

NORTH STAFFORDSHIRE HEALTH AUTHORITY   UNIT No...................

Forms of Consent for Operative Treatment

CONSENT BY PATIENT

I.. of ....

hereby consent to undergo the operation of...

the effect and nature of which have been explained to me.

I also consent to such further alternative operative measures as may be found to be necessary during the course of such operation and to the administration of a local or other anaesthetic for the purpose of the same.

I understand that an assurance has not been given that the operation will be performed by a particular surgeon.

Dated this..............................day of...19......

Signed..

I confirm that I have explained to the patient
the nature and effect of this treatment. Date........................ **Signed**..............................

CONSENT BY RELATIVES

I.. of ....

the...........................of the above named...hereby
also consent to such operation.

Dated this..............................day of...19......

Signed..

I confirm that I have explained the nature and
effect of this operation to the next of kin. Date........................ **Signed**..............................

CONSENT FOR MINOR

I.. of ....

hereby consent to the submission of my child...to

the operation of...the effect and nature of which have

been explained to me.

I also consent to such further alternative operative measures as may be found to be necessary during the course of such operation and to the administration of a local or other anaesthetic for the purpose of the same.
I understand that an assurance has not been given that the operation will be performed by a particular surgeon.

Dated this..............................day of...19......

.... Signed...............................

I confirm that I have explained the nature and effect of this
operation to the child's parent/guardian Date........................ **Signed**..............................

CONSENT FOR E.C.T.

I.. of ....
hereby consent to the administration of convulsive therapy, the effect and nature of which have been explained to me. Notwithstanding the fact that there are certain risks of injury inherent in the treatment, I request you to administer the same to me and I accept any risk attaching to such administration.

I understand that an assurance has not been given that the treatment will be administered by a particular practitioner.

Dated this..............................day of...19......

Signed..

I confirm that I have explained to the patient
the nature and effect of this operation. Date........................ **Signed**..............................

When completed this document should be placed with the case papers of the patient

MR. 21   D. & Co. Ltd.

DEPARTMENT OF GASTROENTEROLOGY

Telephone
Stoke-on-Trent 621133

GASTROINTESTINAL ENDOSCOPY

City General Hospital
Stoke-on-Trent
ST4 6QG

M/S	SURNAME		HOSP	WARD/DEPT	Date	
FIRST NAMES		CONSULTANT				
REG. No			DATE OF BIRTH		Examination	
ADDRESS						
GP's NAME & INITIALS					Instrument	

Provisional Diagnosis	
Reason for Examination	

Drugs Used	Premedication	
	Anaesthetic	
	Other	

	Photographs	Biopsies
Oesophagus		
Stomach		
Duodenum		
Rectum		
Sigmoid and Descending colon		
Transverse and Ascending colon		
Other Procedures		
Comments :		

Copy for patient's notes

Copy for General Practitioner

Copy for Department Files

NORTH STAFFORDSHIRE HEALTH AUTHORITY

WARD			
			Conc. Code Colour

PRESCRIPTION SHEET

Surname	First Names	Hospital Number

Date of Admission			Date of Discharge			N.H.S. Number
Day	Month	Year	Day	Month	Year	

DETAILS OF PREVIOUS MEDICATION

Drug	Dose	Directions	Duration of Treatment

ONCE ONLY AND PREMEDICATION DRUGS
(Continuation Pages Available)

Date	Time	Drug	Dose	Route	Dr's Initials	Time Given	Given By	Pharmacy Use	Code
1									
2									
3									
5									
6									
7									
8									
9									
10									
11									
12									
13									
14									
15									
16									

GENERAL INSTRUCTIONS FOR PRESCRIBERS (Instructions for Nursing Staff on back page)

1. Use Approved Names, BLOCK LETTERS, Metric Dosage and English Instructions.
2. ANY CHANGES in your drug therapy MUST be ordered by a NEW PRESCRIPTION, do NOT alter existing instructions.
3. DISCONTINUE a drug by drawing a line, through both the prescription and the unused recording panels. Enter the date of cancellation in the column provided.
4. Prescribe the intravenous drip therapy, dialysis therapy and anticoagulant therapy on the separate charts provided. An indication that such therapy is being administered should be entered on this sheet.

INDEX